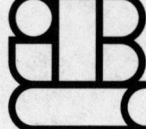

Improving Clinical Practice

Improving Clinical Practice

David Blumenthal, M.D., M.P.P.
Ann C. Scheck, M.S.
Editors

Improving Clinical Practice

Total Quality Management and the Physician

Jossey-Bass Publishers • San Francisco

Substantial discounts on bulk quantities of Jossey-Bass books are available to corporations, professional associations, and other organizations. For details and discount information, contact the special sales department at Jossey-Bass Inc., Publishers.
(415) 433–1740; Fax (800) 605–2665.

For sales outside the United States, please contact your local Paramount Publishing International Office.

 Manufactured in the United States of America on Lyons Falls Pathfinder Tradebook. This paper is acid-free and 100 percent totally chlorine-free.

Library of Congress Cataloging-in-Publication Data

Improving clinical practice: total quality management and the
    physician/David Blumenthal and Ann Scheck, editors.
        p.   cm.
    Includes bibliographical references and index.
    ISBN 0-7879-0093-1
    1. Hospital care–Quality control.   2. Total quality management.
    3. Medical care–Decision making.   4. Hospitals–Medical staff.
    I. Blumenthal, David, 1948–   .   II. Scheck, Ann.
    RA972.I47   1995
    362.1'068'5–dc20   95-3749

FIRST EDITION
HB Printing   10 9 8 7 6 5 4 3 2 1

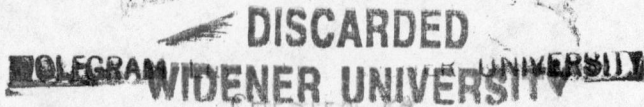

Contents

Preface

This volume has its origins in my personal experience and in some observations about the state of current research on quality management in U.S. health care. As is so often the case, personal experience was in many ways the more compelling force.

From 1987 to 1991, I was Senior Vice President of Brigham and Women's Hospital (BWH), a 720-bed Harvard teaching hospital located adjacent to the Harvard Medical School campus. On arrival in 1987, I was given responsibility for designing a new quality management system for the hospital, a project I embraced with naive enthusiasm. The Brigham and Women's Hospital's interest in quality management did not reflect any unease with the quality of care provided or with the hospital's competitive position; both were regarded as strong and improving. Rather, the impetus for this assignment seemed to lie in a general sense that no matter how good things were, they could be made better. Also, BWH had a close relationship with Harvard Community Health Plan (HCHP), the Boston health maintenance organization, whose staff were experimenting with quality improvement techniques as part of its own, far-sighted competitive thrust in the Eastern Massachusetts marketplace. Efforts by HCHP's management and physicians to improve quality of care raised the sensitivity of BWH's management to the possibility that new and improved methods for ensuring quality of care might be developed.

Together with Dr. Glenn Laffel, a BWH-trained cardiologist hired to lead our quality improvement effort, I began a voyage of discovery that was to affect profoundly my views not only of quality management but also of organizational behavior, human nature, and the functioning of national economies. The voyage began with a careful effort, spearheaded by Laffel, to review existing approaches to quality assurance at the time. We familiarized ourselves with the work of the eminent scholars who had laid the foundation for quality assurance in medicine before and during the mid-1980s: Donabedian, Williamson, Brook, and Chassin. We invited a stream of consultants to describe their approaches and products: automated protocols for reviewing process of care and severity of illness algorithms that facilitated outcome measurement. We also traveled to Nashville, where Dr. Paul Batalden and his staff generously described their plans for improving quality of care in the facilities of the Hospital Corporation of America (HCA). Without false modesty, I can say that we completely missed the import of what Batalden and his colleagues—pioneers in the application of total quality management (TQM)—were attempting to accomplish from their base in HCA's elegant central offices.

The primary product of this educational process was the conviction that, despite the talent and wisdom of the many individuals working in the field of quality assurance, no system existed that we wanted to emulate. We went to the leading edge of quality management in the United States during the mid-1980s and discovered that the field stopped far short of a comprehensive and exciting vision for making quality better and far short of an applied technology that could substitute for the traditional techniques of case review (morbidity and mortality rounds, clinico-pathological conferences, and physician education) that prevailed in our institution and in most others at the time.

In the spring of 1987, I arranged to be invited to a meeting at the Institute of Medicine in Washington, D.C., on the subject of technology assessment. I had few hopes that the conference would make a major difference in my understanding of quality management, but I wanted to be thorough. Milling in the crowd of guests and speakers during a break, I ran into Don Berwick, a longtime friend who was leading the effort to develop a quality assurance system for HCHP. Laffel and I had been in touch with Berwick during our previous research on quality management, and he had shared some very careful, innovative work on quality measurement that he had been conducting within HCHP.

Berwick was much less interested in the conference than he was in describing another event he had just attended. He had stopped in Washington on his way back from four days at a "Deming seminar," his first exposure to the thinking of W. Edwards Deming. Normally calm and contained, Berwick radiated an excitement bordering on elation as he described his experience. Anything that could do that to Don Berwick, I decided, was worth checking out myself.

In October 1987, Laffel and I traveled to Montreal to attend our own Deming seminar. Then eighty-seven, Deming was recovering from a hospitalization at Georgetown University Medical Center, where he had been treated for deep vein thrombophlebitis in a lower extremity. Although he was required to sit with his leg elevated (instead of prowling the stage as he normally did), his teaching on the theory and methods of TQM had the same compelling effect on us as it did on Berwick and so many other attendees from diverse industries and organizations. He also shared with me after the seminar an amusing but perceptive commentary he had written while lying in his hospital bed. It documented vividly the flaws in the processes of care during his recent hospitalization: problems that I knew from personal experience to be endemic in all large health care organizations. This was for me the first evidence that his analytical methods might have applicability to the world of health care organizations.

TQM appealed to me at many levels. As a theory of management, it was humane, democratic, and oriented toward learning and education. Perhaps most important of all, however, it seemed to me grounded fundamentally in the scientific method. TQM advocated the application of validated data, sound statistical analysis, and the experimental method to diagnosing and treating problems in the processes that organizations use to produce their products. As a physician, this is how I had been trained to think about diagnosing and treating problems in my patients' biological processes. The fit seemed natural. The contribution of TQM, I later came to realize, had little to do with the novelty of its analytical techniques or methods. Rather, Deming and other proponents of TQM had developed practical approaches for using the scientific method in daily work. TQM was an applied technology for using science to improve quality. It had to work in a science-based discipline such as medicine.

During the next several years, Laffel and I collaborated with an expanding group of hospital managers and employees to adapt the theory and methods of TQM to improving the quality of care at Brigham and Women's Hospital. We enjoyed a number of successes and experienced numerous setbacks. From my personal standpoint, however, one of the most puzzling problems we encountered early on was our inability to attract the interest or support of any substantial number of physicians in the organization. This failing occurred despite the fact that many of the physicians at BWH were academicians—faculty members at Harvard Medical School—who had devoted their lives and careers to using the scientific method to improve clinical services. How could they not see the promise of TQM for improving patient care?

Over time, I formulated several hypotheses about the relative disinterest of my physician colleagues in TQM. During darker moods, I wondered whether physicians were simply an ornery and backward lot, inherently opposed to new and different ideas. This was, I concluded, neither a useful nor accurate characterization of my colleagues at BWH.

Perhaps, then, I was simply not very good at making the case for using TQM in health care organizations. This might very well have been true, but it did not explain something else I was discovering: many of my physician colleagues trying to introduce TQM at other organizations were encountering similar difficulties in enlisting the enthusiastic support of physician staff.

This finding suggested that the problem lay deeper, and a different hypothesis emerged, a hypothesis that lies at the center of this volume. Perhaps part of the difficulty with involving large numbers of physicians in implementing TQM reflected a legitimate skepticism over whether its methods could be applied to the work they regard as their own: the work of making individual decisions about the care of individual patients. The more I thought about this, the more sense it made. I realized that advocates of TQM had yet to demonstrate how this vast, powerful body of knowledge could be harnessed to improve the diagnosis and treatment of illness by physicians. Indeed, no vocabulary really existed for translating the concepts of TQM—customer orientation, the process as the unit of analysis, the flowchart and the fish-bone diagram, the PDCA cycle—into the language of the physician—presenting complaint, history and physical exam, laboratory and radiological testing, differential diagnosis, treatment, and side effects. Until this verbal bridge was built, and until the applicability of TQM to physicians' work could be demonstrated, the possibility remained that physicians would continue to see the tenets of modern quality theory as fundamentally foreign. It might be useful, but not to what they do, and what they do (at least in their own view) is what medicine is all about.

Whether this hypothesis explained my personal experience at BWH or not, it struck me as a useful topic to explore further, not the least because I was and am convinced that the methods of modern quality management can be used by physicians to improve their care of patients. The purpose of this volume is to investigate precisely this topic: the applicability of modern quality management methods to improving clinical decision making by physicians and other health care personnel involved in the day-to-day care of the well and the ill. In the process of designing the conference that produced the chapters in the volume and in assembling them for publication, my original goal of trying to crack the nut of physician participation in TQM has come to seem much less important. Instead, I have become increasingly intrigued with the much more fundamental question of whether the practice of medicine can be improved through the use of TQM, just as so many other processes of production and service have been improved. I will leave it to the reader to judge whether the work presented here and the promise of TQM justify further investigation of this concept.

A second line of thought and observation also contributed to the development of this volume. Since the mid-1980s, when the concepts of TQM first made their way into health care, the amount of health services research relevant to improving quality of health care has grown enormously. Funded by the federal government and private foundations, this work has resulted in an array of new tools and approaches to quality improvement. These include outcomes research and outcomes management, clinical epidemiology, the development and dissemination of guidelines, critical paths, patient-centered care, approaches to shared decision making by patients and physicians, and the development of improved information systems to assist physician decision making. Gifted investigators have devoted their careers to the development of one or more of these approaches to quality management. Several of these methods have received endorsements of one kind or another from public and private parties. The development and dissemination of guidelines has become an important function of the Agency for Health Care Policy and Research, with strong funding and support from Congress. The collection and dissemination of data about outcomes of care have become a central feature of quality monitoring in New York and Pennsylvania and were used until recently by the Health Care Financing Administration through its annual release of data on mortality rates among Medicare beneficiaries in the nation's hospitals. The Clinton administration's health care reform proposal, the Health Security Act, proposed a comprehensive policy of outcomes monitoring as part of its blueprint for revamping the health care system.

Despite all of this work, however, the accumulating knowledge about quality of care seems at times less than the sum of its parts. Enormous energy is devoted to applying and validating particular technologies, but the technologies seem to stand alone, unrelated to one another. No integrative theory of quality management has emerged that tries to take advantage of the contributions of these diverse, but still disparate, methods.

Health services research and many health services researchers also have shown relatively little interest in TQM. This lack may reflect, in part, the tendency of investigators to focus relentlessly on their own line of work. But my impression is that another factor is at work. A number of researchers have been exposed to TQM in one form or another and have reacted negatively. The reasons for this are undoubtedly numerous, but at least three seem operative.

The first is that proponents of TQM, especially in large seminars, tend to adopt an evangelistic or inspirational tone that is disquieting to scientific investigators. The same phenomenon at times has turned away physicians exposed to TQM. The impression created is that TQM is another in a long line of quasi-religious or cult-like approaches to changing human or organizational behavior and is likely to have just as much validity and staying power.

A second reason for the negative reaction of health services researchers to TQM is that some perceive it to be unfairly dismissive of other approaches to quality management, such as guidelines, outcomes measurement, or traditional efforts to investigate the relationships between process and outcomes of care. Certainly, the tendency among some advocates of TQM has been to underestimate the value and contribution of past scholarship on quality of care and of the programs based on that scholarship.

A third reason for the skepticism of some health services researchers about TQM is that they perceive its methods as simplistic and, therefore, of questionable validity. This concern is apparent in Dr. Sheldon Greenfield's chapter (Chapter Three) in this volume. In some cases, this perception arises from an incomplete exposure to TQM's statistical methods at introductory seminars designed to be comprehensible to audiences with minimal statistical training.

Whatever the reason for the negativity of some health services researchers toward TQM, the phenomenon is both avoidable and regrettable. It is avoidable because it is based on misperceptions and misunderstandings on both sides. Far from a latter day religion or a new form of psychobabble, the concepts and methods of TQM are grounded in the scientific method. No fundamental incompatibility exists between the methods of TQM and the new technologies now under development by health services researchers to improve quality of care; in fact, they should be mutually reinforcing.

Furthermore, it is incorrect to perceive the analytical techniques of TQM as simplistic. True, TQM has simplified certain statistical methods to make them accessible to relatively unsophisticated workers so that they can be used to improve processes of daily work. However, these tools make up in utility what they may lose in accuracy. In many ways, the statistical methods of TQM are best understood as supporting what statisticians call "exploratory data analysis." Such analysis is meant to suggest hypotheses, not to accept or reject them, and to lay the basis for further study (confirmatory data analysis) that is more definitive.

The skepticism of many health services researchers toward TQM is regrettable as well. The reason is that TQM potentially could provide a helpful framework to integrate and coordinate the many discrete technologies now under development for the purpose of improving quality of care and service in the health care industry.

The body of knowledge applied in TQM is the most complete theoretical and practical guide to understanding and improving quality that currently exists. As early as the 1950s, textbooks on total quality control and total quality management anticipated virtually all of the basic technologies now under development in the health industry to improve quality of care and service. The current interest in measuring outcomes of care is anticipated in TQM's unwavering commitment to measuring quality for the purpose of improving it. The modern enthusiasm for guidelines, algorithms, and critical paths in health care is anticipated by TQM's use of flow-charts to guide and reduce variability in the process of production and service in industrial organizations. The idea that patients' perceptions can provide valid data on quality of health care is presaged by a central tenet of TQM: quality consists of meeting the needs and expectations of the consumer. (W. Edwards Deming had a stint as a marketing researcher doing surveys for advertising firms on Madison Avenue during the 1940s. He was well acquainted, therefore, with the importance of consumer perceptions of quality to the success of industrial organizations.)

The completeness and usefulness of TQM's precepts do not reflect divine inspiration or supernatural wisdom on the part of Walter Shewhart, Joseph Juran, W. Edwards Deming, or the other thinkers—now glorified almost to excess—who contributed to TQM's development. Rather, the contribution of TQM is the product of decades of refinement through experience in multiple industries and countries.

In fact, what is now called "total quality management" had very humble beginnings in efforts by statisticians at the turn of the century to improve the detection of defective telephones as they came off the assembly line at Western Electric's New York plant. During the next several decades, the work of quality theorists was concerned predominantly with perfecting these statistical methods and concepts—now called "sampling theory"—and making their ideas accessible to workers on assembly lines; thus, the Shewhart control chart. During World War II, quality managers from Bell Labs (where Western Electric's quality theorists came to rest) were detailed to the proving grounds of the U.S. military, where they applied their ideas to improving U.S. weapons and ordnance. After World War II, on the basis of experiences with the widespread use of scientific methods of quality improvement in Japan, a new group of quality theorists began to see quality improvement in a broader context. They came to appreciate that the successful application of the scientific method within industries often required changes in human attitudes and behaviors, including changes in the style of management within organizations. This recognition led Feigenbaum[1] to elaborate the concept of total quality control in the early 1950s. Deming, Juran, Ishikawa, and Crosby expanded on these ideas. In many ways, their teachings reflect the distilled wisdom of thousands of experiences with trying to assist living, breathing, fallible human beings to become more scientific in their approach to improving quality.

The fundamental source of the power of TQM lies in this simultaneous commitment to the scientific method on the one hand and to applying that method in real-world settings on the other. The result is a remarkable blending and interaction of theory and practice that is now available to physicians and other health care practitioners interested in taking advantage of it. The purpose of this volume is to make the connections between TQM and the daily work of physicians more apparent and thereby to potentiate the work of quality managers, clinicians, and researchers in improving quality of care and service in health care organizations.

Overview of the Contents

To approach this ambitious task, the volume is divided into three general parts. In the first part, attempts are made to lay a conceptual basis for the applicability of TQM to the work of physicians and to the community of mainstream health services researchers who continue to pioneer new methods for quality improvement. In Chapter One, Dr. Donald Berwick describes various diverse scientific methodologies that TQM attempts to integrate into a useful package of applied technologies. In this discussion, Berwick makes clear that the foundations of TQM rest not on religious faith, but on empirical methods and inductive reasoning that have been developed and applied during many decades of trial and error. In the second chapter, which appeared in much condensed and modified form in the *Journal of the American Medical Association*, I explore the history and evolution of TQM generally and the potential applicability of certain statistical tools used by TQM to the management of individual patients by individual physicians. In Chapter Three, Dr. Sheldon Greenfield poses a warning for practitioners of TQM. One of the fathers of outcomes research and one of the most widely respected researchers on new quality methods, Greenfield notes that both physicians and health services researchers are skeptical of TQM because of its apparent tendency to dismiss the value of preceding work on health care quality and because of the apparent lack of sophistication of certain commonly used TQM techniques, including the control chart. Nevertheless, Greenfield sees the potential for complementarity between the fields of outcomes research and TQM. In the concluding chapter of this first part (Chapter Four), Albert Mulley draws out the potential for synergy between outcomes research and TQM by exploring more directly their similarities and differences and their tendency to focus on improving quality at different points in the process of patient care.

The second part of the book has a more practical, clinical focus. Its three chapters explore the applicability of TQM to improving clinical decision making and practice in particular disease contexts. Two of these involve hypertension, which is by far the most common clinical malady to afflict the population of the industrial world and which fills the days of the typical primary care practitioner. In Chapter Five, Duncan Neuhauser, Dr. Linda Headrick, and their colleagues discuss some pilot work they have done in using control charts to help patients and doctors manage antihypertensive medications in daily care. Dr. Glenn Laffel discusses more generally (in Chapter Six) the potential applicability of TQM to the management of hypertension. He draws on current understanding of the physiology and regulation of blood pressure in humans to demonstrate how the techniques of TQM may assist with monitoring and controlling blood pressure. In the last chapter in Part Two (Chapter Seven), Dr. Brent James recounts the way he has used TQM to shed light on how the operative management of benign prostatic hypertrophy may be improved. Here, we see the potential applicability of TQM at the detailed level of improving surgical technique.

In the third and concluding part of the volume, the focus shifts to the opportunities and obstacles facing practitioners of TQM who are interested in involving physicians in their work. In two chapters in this section, empirical work on the current participation of physicians in quality management using TQM techniques is discussed. In Chapter Eight, Stephen Shortell and his colleagues discuss the results of surveys and case studies performed in a sample of hospitals in the Western United States. His work is the only systematic, quantitative exploration of this topic and leads to recommendations for making TQM work in health care organizations. And in the following chapter (Chapter Nine), Jennifer Edwards and I describe the results of case studies conducted in six health care organizations with reputations for leadership in quality management using TQM techniques. Our work overlaps with and reinforces the conclusions of Shortell and his colleagues. Dr. John Ball, for more than a decade the executive director of the American College of Physicians, and I broaden the discussion still further to the question of public policy and its effects on physician involvement in TQM. Our chapter (Chapter Ten) is a sobering reflection on the many challenges that are beyond the immediate control of health care organizations but that heavily affect their ability to involve their physicians in the vital work of quality improvement. Finally, in Chapter Eleven, I reflect on the potential value of TQM in helping physicians to realize their aspirations to make their care of patients more scientific, and to enhance the public's regard for them as professionals.

Acknowledgments

For assistance with this volume, Ann Scheck and I are indebted to numerous organizations, groups, and individuals. First and foremost is the Robert Wood Johnson Foundation, whose generous funding made possible the conference at which most of these chapters originally were presented (from October 3 to 5, 1993, in Hanover, New Hampshire) and the research that underlies Chapter Eight, "Physician Involvement in Quality Improvement." I am especially indebted to Alan Cohen, then Vice President of the foundation, who originally encouraged this work, and to Beth Stevens, Senior Program Officer, who provided continuing advice and guidance.

As co-organizer of the conference and the project's original co-investigator, Jennifer Edwards deserves special credit for her insights, thoroughness, patience, and dedication to detail. This work would not have been possible without her assistance. The organization of the conference in New Hampshire also benefited greatly from the advice and experience of David Helms, President of the Alpha Center, whose staff helped run the proceedings.

Stephen Shortell not only contributed enormously through his scholarly work but also collaborated directly on the case study of the Intermountain Health System. I learned a tremendous amount about how to conduct case studies from watching his thorough and insightful methods. Dr. Jack Wennberg and his colleagues at Dartmouth, as informal hosts, helped make the conference in Hanover both relaxed and productive.

Dawn DaCosta and Anne Fulton provided invaluable administrative support in organizing the conference and in producing this volume. I am also continually indebted to Massachusetts General Hospital—Dr. John Potts, its Chief of Medicine, and Dr. Albert Mulley, Chief of General Internal Medicine, for their encouragement and support.

Finally, I want to thank my wife, Dr. Ellen Blumenthal, who puts up with me through thick and thin.

March 1995   David Blumenthal, M.D., M.P.P.
                                                        Boston, Massachusetts

Notes

1. Feigenbaum, A. V. (1983). *Total Quality Control* (3rd ed.). New York: McGraw-Hill.

About the Authors

John R. Ball, M.D., J.D., is currently Senior Scholar at the Association of Academic Health Centers. He earned his M.D. and J.D. degrees from Duke University. For the past thirteen years, he has been associated with the American College of Physicians (ACP): first as Associate Executive Vice President for Health and Public Policy and then as Executive Vice President (1986–1994). Prior to joining ACP, Dr. Ball spent three years in the Public Health Service and three years as Senior Policy Analyst in the Office of Science and Technology Policy in the Carter White House. He is a member of the Institute of Medicine, the board of managers of the Pennsylvania Hospital, and the board of directors of the Milbank Memorial Fund. His substantive policy interests have been the medical work force, quality assurance, technology assessment, and the role of the professional society.

Donald M. Berwick, M.D., M.P.P., is President and CEO of the Institute for Healthcare Improvement, a nonprofit organization dedicated to helping accelerate the pace of improvement of the health care systems of the United States and Canada. He is a practicing pediatrician at the Harvard Community Health Plan, Associate Professor of Pediatrics at the Harvard Medical School, and Adjunct Associate Professor of Health Policy and Management at the Harvard School of Public Health. Dr. Berwick serves as Vice-Chair of the Preventive Services Task Force of the U.S. Department of Health and Human Services, and from 1989 through 1991 was a member of the Panel of Judges of the Malcolm Baldrige National Quality Award Program. He serves on the board of directors of the Juran Institute. He holds a bachelor's degree summa cum laude from Harvard College, a master's degree in public policy from the John F. Kennedy School of Government, and an M.D. from Harvard Medical School.

David Blumenthal, M.D., M.P.P., is Chief of the Health Policy Research and Development Unit and Associate Physician at the Massachusetts General Hospital in Boston. He is also Associate Professor of Medicine and Associate Professor of Health Care Policy at Harvard Medical School. From 1987 to 1991, he was Senior Vice President at Boston's Brigham and Women's Hospital, a 720-bed Harvard teaching hospital. In 1988, he served as chief health adviser to the Dukakis presidential campaign. From 1981 to 1987, he was Executive Director of the Center for Health Policy and Management and Lecturer on Public Policy at the John F. Kennedy School of Government at Harvard. During the late 1970s, Dr. Blumenthal was a professional staff member on Senator Edward Kennedy's Senate Subcommittee on Health and Scientific Research. He is a member of several editorial boards, including the *New England Journal of Medicine, Inquiry, Quality Management in Health Care,* and the *Bulletin of the New York Academy of Medicine,* and serves on advisory committees to the National Academy of Sciences, the Institute of Medicine, the U.S. Office of Technology Assessment, and several foundations. His research interests include quality management in health care, the determinants of physician behavior, access to health services, and the extent and consequences of academic-industrial relationships in the health sciences.

Jennifer N. Edwards, Dr.P.H., M.H.S., is Director of the Bureau of Ambulatory Care at the Massachusetts Rate Setting Commission.

The Rate Setting Commission provides data and policy analysis to health care providers, purchasers, and policymakers in the commonwealth. She was previously a Research Associate at Massachusetts General Hospital's Health Policy Research and Development Unit. Her research interests include the application of data to improve health care delivery systems and access to care for vulnerable populations. She received her doctoral degree from the Pew Health Policy Program, University of Michigan.

Sheldon Greenfield, M.D., is an internist, having completed his residency at the Beth Israel Hospital in Boston, where he began work on clinical algorithms for nurse practitioners in the early 1970s. His pioneering research on guidelines has been not only for nurse practitioners but also for use in quality of care assessment by chart audit and, most recently, for physicians. With his Boston colleagues, he performed a series of randomized, controlled trials comparing nurse practitioners using algorithms to physicians, with respect to patient outcomes. He then turned to quality of care measurement, devising a method called "criteria mapping," which applies branching logic and decision making to retrospective chart review, using outcomes to validate the method. In recent years, he has worked with others to increase patient participation in care by using patient-oriented guidelines and by using outcomes to determine the value of that participation. He is currently Medical Director of the Medical Outcome Study (MOS), which seeks to compare systems of care, specialties, various aspects of interpersonal care, and resource use to outcome and, in that position, has become one of the leading clinician outcomes researchers in the country. He is Principal Investigator of the Type II diabetes patient outcome research team (PORT). He was Chairman of the Quality of Care Committee at UCLA for some years and was a Co-Director of the RAND UCLA Center for Health Policy Study. He is former President of the Society of General Internal Medicine. He recently completed a four-year tenure as Chairman of the Health Care Technology Study Section for the Agency for Health Care Policy and Research.

Brent C. James, M.D., M.Stat., Executive Director of the IHC Institute for Health Care Delivery Research and Assistant Vice President for Medical Research, is board certified in general surgery. He is an Adjunct Assistant Professor in the Division of Biostatistics, Department of Family and Preventive Medicine, University of Utah Medical Center, Salt Lake City, and a Visiting Lecturer in the Department of Biostatistics, Harvard School of Public Health, where he was an Assistant Professor in the Department of Biostatistics and a biostatistician with the Eastern Cooperative Oncology Group. His publication *Quality Management for Health Care Delivery* describes the application of continuous quality improvement to clinical medicine.

Glenn L. Laffel, M.D., Ph.D., recently joined APM, Inc., as a Senior Clinical Consultant. He is recognized internationally for his work on the health care applications of total quality management. Recently, he has focused on related fields, such as clinical resource management, physician-hospital collaboration, and managed care readiness. He is the founding editor of *Quality Management in Health Care*, a journal dedicated to rigorous analysis of the quality movement in this industry. This year, he served as a judge for the Commitment to Quality Award. Dr. Laffel has worked with many U.S. health care organizations, including the Institute for Healthcare Improvement, the Healthcare Forum, the School of Public Health at Harvard, the University of Maryland Medical System, the Vanderbilt Institute for Public Policy, Cedars Sinai Medical Center, Monmouth Medical Center, the Mid-Maine Medical Center, the American Society for Quality Control, and the National Association of Children's Hospitals and Related Institutions. He has spoken in eleven countries on subjects referable to quality management. Formerly, he was Director of Quality Management at Brigham and Women's Hospital in Boston. In addition, he is a cardiologist with special interests in the area of heart transplantation. Dr. Laffel received a bachelor's degree in biology and psychology from Tufts University, where he graduated with magna cum laude honors. He received his M.D. from the University of Miami

School of Medicine, where he was elected to Alpha Omega Alpha, the medical honors society. He received his doctoral degree in health policy and management from the Massachusetts Institute of Technology.

Albert G. Mulley, Jr., M.D., is Associate Professor of Medicine and Associate Professor of Health Policy at Harvard Medical School and Chief of the General Internal Medicine Division and Director of the Medical Practices Evaluation Center at Massachusetts General Hospital. After receiving degrees in medicine and public policy from Harvard, he completed his residency training in internal medicine at Massachusetts General Hospital. He is author and editor of the text *Primary Care Medicine* and of many articles in the medical and health services research literature. Dr. Mulley's recent research has focused on the use of decision analysis, outcomes research, and preference assessment methods to distinguish between warranted and unwarranted variations in clinical practice. This work has led to development of research instruments and approaches, including shared decision-making programs using interactive videodisc technology to inform patients about treatment options and to catalyze large-scale prospective clinical trials.

Duncan Neuhauser, Ph.D., is Professor of Epidemiology and Biostatistics, Professor of Medicine, Professor of Family Medicine, and Keck Foundation Research Scholar. He is a Professor of Organizational Behavior and Co-Director of Health Systems Management in the Weatherhead School of Management. All of these appointments are at Case Western University, Cleveland, Ohio. He is an adjunct member of the medical staff of Cleveland Metro Health Center, Cleveland Clinic Foundation, and University Hospitals of Cleveland. He is editor of *Medical Care* and a member of the Institute of Medicine. He received his doctoral degree in business administration from the University of Chicago in 1971. His research interest is in the organization of management of health care, cost-effective clinical decision analysis, ongoing patient randomization, and clinical process improvement.

Ann C. Scheck, M.S., is a doctoral candidate in Health Policy and Management at the Harvard School of Public Health. She is also an independent consultant to a variety of health care organizations and has evaluated programs for the World Health Organization, developed a TQM program for a teaching hospital in Bogota, Columbia, and worked for a variety of not-for-profit health care systems and hospitals in the United States. From 1987 1990, Ms. Scheck worked in the health care industry in Los Angeles, as a consultant with Arthur Young & Company, and as a manager at the University of California, Los Angeles Medical Center. Her current projects include research on access to care and satisfaction with care among differently insured populations, cost-effectiveness analysis of knee surgery options, and developing a workers' compensation outcomes management program for a health care system in California that incorporates quality management principles. Scheck received her bachelor's and master's degrees with distinction and honors from Stanford University.

Stephen M. Shortell, Ph.D., is the A. C. Buehler Distinguished Professor of Health Services Management and Professor of Organization Behavior in the Department of Organization Behavior at the J. L. Kellogg Graduate School of Management, Northwestern University, Evanston, Illinois. He also holds appointments in the School of Medicine at Northwestern and is a member of the Center for Health Services and Policy Research. Dr. Shortell received his bachelor's degree from the University of Notre Dame, his master's degree in public health and hospital administration from the University of California at Los Angeles, and his doctoral degree in the behavioral sciences from the University of Chicago. A leading health care scholar, Dr. Shortell is the senior author of *Strategic Change in Turbulent Times*, which received the George R. Terry Book of the Year Award from the Academy of Management for its contributions to management knowledge. His most recent co-edited book, *Improving Health Policy and Management*, received the James R. Hamilton Book of the Year Award from the American College of Healthcare Executives. He also has been the recipient of both the Dean Conley and Edgar G. Hayhow Article of the Year Awards from the American College of Healthcare Executives. He is an elected member of the Institute of Medicine of the National Academy of Sciences; has served as President of the Association for Health Services Research; and has served as Chairman of the Accrediting Commission for Graduate Education in Health Services Administration. He currently is conducting research on the strategy, structure, and performance of integrated health systems and is assessing the implementation and impact of continuous quality improvement/total quality management on U.S. health care organizations.

Improving Clinical Practice

PART ONE

Concepts

1

Improving as Science

Donald M. Berwick, M.D., M.P.P.

The Problem

It was a typical day in the office. Jim, my fifth patient of the after-noon, needed a tuberculin test, according to his principal, before he could be enrolled; dutifully, I placed it on his arm. The system for reporting the result was standard: wait seventy-two hours and then have the patient feel the site of the skin test for a lump, check off on the preprinted, embossed postcard the box that most closely corresponds to the size of the lump (in a normal child, one hopes there would be no lump at all), and mail the card back to me for entry into Jim's record. Simple.

I reached into the bin of preprinted cards in the examination room. Empty. Undaunted, I headed into the reception area to the master bin to refill the examining room stock. Empty.

At some time in every busy doctor's day, a particular sound begins to roll like ominous, approaching thunder. It is the sound of the charts of waiting patients dropping into the Lucite bins on examining room doors. Thunk, thunk, thunk . . . . It is the sound of more and more work undone that, as the day progresses, gradually becomes the undoing of the doctor. The backlog grows, and I expe-rience the feeling of that recurring dream most have in which we must run but our legs will not move.

All I need is a little white card; it is all that stands between me and the next patient. But the bin is empty. The bin is always empty.

I reach my limit, and in pain I take the only action I know how to take after four years of college, four of medical school, three of residency, one of fellowship, and fifteen of practice. I scream, "Charlie!"

Charlie comes. He is my clinical assistant, and he was trained in heaven. "What's wrong, doctor?" he asks. Wordless, I point with jabbing fingers toward the empty box of cards, my lips quivering. As always, Charlie understands.

He takes me by the hand and leads me back through the inner sanctum of the utility room into a large walk-in closet, which he unlocks with a key. With a second key, he unlocks a cabinet in the closet and removes a large, olive green, metal box from the cabinet. He unlocks the box with a third key, opens it, reaches his hand under a sheaf of papers, and holds before me a stack of one hundred—maybe two hundred—pristine, white, preprinted tuberculin test cards.

"I hid these," says Charlie, smiling. "You can have one."

If we had not been cramped into a utility room closet, I might have kissed Charlie and danced with him there on the spot. "Oh, thank you, thank you," I purred. Once again, Charlie had saved the day.

"Why did you hide these?" I asked.

"I have to," he said. "We run out of them all the time because (and here he scowled) Internal Medicine comes and steals them."

Now I come to the question that must concern us. The question is this: is Charlie—my savior in this story—a hero? Or is he a goat? Rather, because Charlie is definitely not, in any molecule of his being, a goat, the question can be reframed: in this story, is Charlie helping solve the American health care crisis? Or is he, in part, causing it?

Think about that as I relate a second story that also will give us grist for these ideas.

This is a story about David, twelve years old and in the hospital, with me as his attending physician, because his kidneys failed temporarily as a result of post-streptococcal glomerulonephritis. David's main complication was inappropriate fluid balance, leading to hypertension that, though asymptomatic, could further damage his kidneys and cause other troubles. Our job—mine and the house staff's—was to control his hypertension while his kidneys recovered.

Here is how we controlled his hypertension. During his nine days in the hospital, we asked the nurses to measure David's blood pressure. They did; according to the records, they did it 216 times in nine days, using three different measurement methods: an intraarterial catheter connected to a pressure gauge, a standard inflatable blood pressure cuff, and a doppler flow detection device. "They" included nurses, LPNs, and pediatric residents on three different shifts and in two different hospital wards, because David was transferred on the fourth day of his stay. His 216 blood pressures readings were recorded in tabular form, along with pulse rates, temperatures, scattered nursing notes, and medication records, on seventeen different sheets of paper.

To control David's blood pressure, his doctors used four different medications—one of them (nifedipine) administered by two different routes, oral and sublingual. It is difficult to reconstruct David's 216 hours of care from the existing written record, but if "adjustment" of treatment is defined to mean any change in the type, dose, route, or schedule of a medicine, I would estimate conservatively that David's antihypertensive treatment was "adjusted" fifty-four times during his stay, by eleven people, in response to 216 measurements of blood pressure and pulse.

That is a relatively complex system of stimulus and response. It all ended for the hospital on the day David went home—to the care of his local doctor—with his hypertension, we might assume, exquisitely controlled by a perfect combination of furosemide, oral nifedipine, and sublingual nifedipine. His discharge note read, in relevant part: "medications: Lasix 20 mgm, p.o. bid; nifedipine 20 mgm, p.o. bid; nifedipine 5 mgm, s.l. prn."

On closer scrutiny, however, this finely honed system appears to have some problems. First, David's discharge order does not correspond to any of the fifty-four treatment plans that were used during his hospital stay. Second, the sublingual nifedipine capsules of five milligrams that were used on occasional nights during his hospitalization are specially fabricated by the hospital pharmacy for inpatient use and are nowhere available "on the outside" to either David or his local doctor. Third, given David's return home and the consequent inevitable major changes in both his diet and activity pattern as compared with his experience in the hospital, it is impossible to find a single involved clinician who believes that David's blood pressure pattern at home or his response to treatment can be predicted successfully by those patterns in the hospital. Fourth, a simple graph of David's blood pressures over time, prepared only after his discharge, shows little or no consistent relationship between David's in-hospital blood pressure pattern and the various treatments used to control it. In fact, it might be fair to call the blood pressure variation statistically "random," showing no perceptible relationship between treatments and level.

I could not imagine a more dedicated crew of doctors, nurses, and technicians in any hospital than those who joined me in caring for David. I feel privileged to know them and proud to share in their professional work. Like Charlie, each is a proud and inventive solver of problems. Each struggles day and night to do his or her very best for David and for every other patient; each, in fact, lives in quiet fear of causing an error in care. Each checks and double-checks the data and considers very carefully the risks and benefits of any treatment. Each makes decisions—tough ones—and each lies sleepless at least some nights, reviewing the day's work and wondering whether those decisions made were the best possible ones.

But, I suggest, in their striving for excellence, the actions of each of those dedicated people caring for David must bring to our minds the same question I asked about Charlie: hero? or goat? Are they really solving problems, or are they causing them?

Let's look deeper; these two stories may provide a foundation for an important and general hypothesis—namely, that we are trapped. All of us are trapped—Charlie, David's care team, health services researchers, and health care providers. We are trapped in a system of care that leaves us torn between our own desires to serve and to excel on the one hand and the legitimate, burning need of our patients and society to perfect the system as a whole on the other.

Let me clarify this concept. In hiding the cards, Charlie excels. Proudly, he meets my need—locally, specifically, in the instant. But within the system, Charlie hinders, destroys. His habit of heroism removes resources from the mainstream, prevents staff in Internal Medicine from getting what they need, insults colleagues (he calls them "thieves"), and most damaging of all, never, never, never can contribute to the permanent improvement of the underlying system of causes. Why, after all, do the cards ever run out at all?

The same, in more subtle ways, applies to David's medical management. Each resident perfects his or her local, immediate decision. Each listens carefully to that night's nurse, reviews that night's records, and makes a considered change in that night's care. But the system as a whole is never constructed. Locally, specifically, in the instant, each decision makes sense; it is the best decision each decision maker can make. It is only when we as team members step back, away from the instance, and view the system of care as the whole of David's experience instead of our individual experiences, that we begin to see the true quantity of waste, variation, and disarray that we have created despite our very best intentions.

One of us raises the dose and the other reduces it, on successive nights, yet both are responding to random variation. One of us believes the other is calling the local doctor, and vice versa; the local doctor complains that no one ever called her. The pharmacist, proudly, prepares a special formula for David's nifedipine, which we, proudly, dispense, but together we have created a treatment plan that is impossible to continue effectively at home the day after tomorrow.

We try our best, succeed locally, and utterly fail as a system. This is our trap.

Science in the Service of Improvement

As a twenty-two-year-old intern at the bedside of Bobby Franklin, a six-year-old with acute lymphoblastic leukemia, I also was trapped. I tried hard to do well, administering fragments of treatment to relieve one symptom at a time—to quell the fever, to restore nutrition, to ease the pain. But I felt, too, the relentless, undeflected, sinister march of the disease system as a whole. Even while struggling as hard as I could hour by hour, I sensed a latent, underlying cause beyond the reach of my fragments of weaponry that in its own inexorable logic mocked my best efforts. Bobby died.

Today, twenty years later, science has disarmed the enemy. In 1995, Bobby would not have died. The history of conquering acute lymphoblastic leukemia is a victory, in part, of knowledge. To beat leukemia required a system of improvement that could set an aim, identify the causal dynamics in a system of interest, set up and conduct informative trials to build on that information, and deploy the knowledge gained within the real system at work: the care of patients. Today, if we as physicians do not understand the linkage between science and the improvement of patient care, we cannot really call ourselves doctors. Knowledge and progress combine, linked by action taken on the basis of knowledge.

But what about Charlie and David? In the stories I related, how effectively do we as doctors link knowledge and action to achieve progress?

Not well at all. Ask Charlie. The question I would put is this: "Charlie, in the future, month after month, do you predict that the need to hide the cards will increase or decrease? You hide the cards to relieve a symptom of a deeper problem. Will that problem go away?"

Charlie would not answer first in words. Instead, he would just laugh, as he asked in reply, "Why would the problem go away? It has always been there, and so I would guess that it will persist."

Similarly, it would be with David. First, "I notice," I said to the junior resident, "that David's medications get changed a lot—probably more than he needs. Why don't we create a graph of his blood pressures over time and analyze the variation more systematically to see what is random change and what is not?"

"That's a great idea," said the resident, "but I leave the service tomorrow, and anyway, it's the nurses who measure the blood pressures."

So I spoke with the head nurse, who also thought it was a good idea. However, it next would have to pass through the hospital's Forms Committee, which only meets every two months. "And, of course," she added, "we'd have to look at the implications for staffing ratios—my nurses are already flat out."

There, as far as I know, the idea died.

Standing outside the system of care, those who watch doctors work are frustrated indeed. What they notice, above all, is that we do not seem to change. Our costs rise steadily. We make them wait. We often do not answer their questions, and we are inconsistent when we do. We quote policies in response to their pain. Instead of meeting their needs, we explain why we cannot do so. We disavow responsibility for the United States ranking twenty-first among developed nations in infant mortality, for having cesarean section rates four times those in Holland, for having an infant mortality rate among African American babies 240 percent higher than among Caucasian babies, and for national health care expenditures 40 percent higher than those of the next most costly nation. The frustration breeds anger, the anger breeds demands, the demands breed controls, and the controls breed reprisals.

I believe it all originates from helplessness—helplessness exactly analogous to the helplessness I felt at Bobby Franklin's bedside, watching him die in the years before discovering the linked knowledge and action that would have made his death avoidable. Those outside the system think doctors do not want to improve the health care system as a whole. The problem, however, is that doctors do not know how.

Classifying the Sciences of System Improvement

Science, linking knowledge to action, beat acute lymphoblastic leukemia. Similarly, science linked to action can help establish the health care system that is needed.

Skepticism is understandable. Some important differences exist between the diseases of the body and the afflictions of a health care system. The former fit more neatly into the framework of science: assays, models, etiologies, and experiments all seem better suited for the problems of tuberculosis or leukemia than they do for waste, inappropriateness, complexity, miscommunication, or indignity. Moreover, although we as doctors can believe in an underlying generalizability for diseases—the tuberculid is the same in my body or yours in most important ways—this does not seem to be as consistently true for interpersonal and organizational systems. What causes senseless variation in David's pharmacotherapy seems to be much more of a local issue—a characteristic of *that* hospital, *that* ward, *those* doctors, and *that* patient—than a general property of such components interacting as a system. Science seeks generalizations; but real systems are each special.[1]

I believe that the central question I am trying to answer is this: What are the relationships between the familiar sciences of biomedicine and clinical care on the one hand and the less familiar sciences through which others have tried to understand and improve complex human and organizational systems on the other?

One premise behind that question is the flat assertion that there *are* sciences through which complex systems can be understood and improved. It is to that assertion that I address the remainder of my comments. I wish to offer a classification of the "sciences of improvement" that we can use to organize our thinking about quality management in clinical care.

That systemic improvement methods can be called "scientific" is itself an assertion that may surprise some. Trained medically, we tend to think of clinical work as "scientific" and managerial work as not "scientific." We link the privilege of caring for patients to mastery of specific knowledge and methods—scientific knowledge and the scientific method. But the privilege of running a system of care—running the health care system—seems linked, not to science, but to rituals, credentials, and structures of influence of which we remain ignorant and often critical.

Here, we call that dichotomy into question. Specifically, we must explore the assertion that "modern management sciences"[5] have matured to a remarkable extent and that they offer us all a way to become more methodical about improving the system in which we give care, and not just the care we give within that system. Even more boldly, we must explore whether these same scientific approaches to systems can contribute usefully to the improvement of individual patient care, heretofore largely the domain of biomedical sciences.

W. Edwards Deming, a statistician and physicist by training and therefore one who knows the language and ritual of science, offers an extremely powerful classification scheme for understanding the sciences relevant to leadership of a system.[2] His is the scheme I follow.

The Science of Understanding Systems

First are sciences relevant to knowledge of the *system as a whole*. The intellectual roots are in general systems theory; important modern contributors include Forrester, Ackoff[3], Bertalanffy[4], and Senge.[5] The common theme in this field is the formal concept of a "system" as, in Ackoff's words, "a set of interdependent parts sharing a common purpose."[6] This simple idea spawns many complicated questions, each of which has kept its full share of academicians busy for decades; for example:

- How can one acquire a view of the system as a whole? We as doctors are accustomed to exploring the world in fragments. When we seek to connect those fragments conceptually, how do we discover which we should include within a system and which should be left outside? Where do we draw boundaries, and why? What system cares for David, and why would we define it as such?

- What are the types or classifications of systems, and how do they differ from one another? One classical dichotomy is between "closed" systems, which are self-referential and tend toward homeostasis, as in a thermostat or in the pituitary-adrenal axis, and "open" systems, which are affected by non-system influences, as happens when I reset a thermostat or when a child learns to read.

- How do nonlinear systems—those with feedback loops and delays, for example—behave? When are they predictable, and when not? How does one find points of special influence or optimal solutions? It is in this inquiry that systems theory has links to the emergent science-of-chaos theory.

- Where do systems find their aims? How do people or elements communicate with each other and with the world outside their system? When a system's purpose is to meet an outside need, how does it explore and understand that need, and then how does it translate understanding into a coordinated effort to meet the need?

- What is the relationship between the part and the whole? Specifically, how does one element of a system support the performance of the system as a whole instead of "suboptimizing" in favor of its own, local performance? Suboptimization in systems terms can be a constant threat to achieving the purpose of the whole.

Scientifically, we can label Charlie's behavior and much of David's care as examples of suboptimization—parts being improved without cognizance, and perhaps even at the expense, of the performance of the system as a whole. Charlie hides cards because he cannot envision or participate effectively in a system in which it would be unnecessary to hide cards. The night float jiggles David's medication because she cannot recognize or participate effectively in an overall strategy for David's pharmacotherapy.

In David's case, systems issues even arise at a more technical level. We know, for example, that the entire system that determines his blood pressure is comprised of a set of interdependent influences. Drugs interact with each other, as well as with his diet, his level of activity, his mood, his parents' behavior, his specific interactions with staff, and even the knowledge and skill of those who measure his blood pressure and write his medication orders. Imagine if we tried to write down each of these factors and then drew arrows of influence showing whether and how each factor affected the other. The page soon would look like a child's scribble—a drawing of a system that appears both daunting and unsolvable.

In fact, such a system *is* unsolvable. Russell Ackoff[3] uses the term *mess* to describe what we would see. A mess is a system of problems in which each problem affects the others. One may adopt the illusion of "solving" one problem or another, but it is in the nature of systems that the mess cannot be solved as a whole. We can adjust tonight's nifedipine, but we cannot "adjust" the system that produces David's blood pressure.

Unfortunately, solving a problem is often a form of suboptimization. The individual problem may be solved, but the mess gets worse. This is the world of the systems thinker, a world in which the effort to understand often walks on the edge of chaos. It is a world of approximation, iteration, synthesis, and connection, not a world of exactitude, solution, analysis, and segmentation. It is a world familiar in the experience of doctors, but not one well supported by the language and culture of professional behaviors. We are supposed to solve problems, but we live in a mess, which is never resolved.

To manage care in a way such that Charlie can interact effectively with the other elements of the system in which he works is a basic aspiration of those who work to improve quality. Furthermore, as long as we cannot work *on* the system, we are doomed to work *in* it. But there is promise here. The sciences of systems could conceivably help us practice better medicine. In David's case, it probably would help if the senior resident were to call a pause in the chase and work with her team to draw the system of influences on David's blood pressure. It would help also if the junior resident had the skill, the time, and the social support to develop a sense of who composed the system of David's care and to ask herself about degrees of precision, integrity, and clarity within those system component interdependencies. An understanding of nonlinearities might help when the medical and nursing teams faced oscillations in their own decisions that produced apparently meaningless cycles of increases, decreases, and increases in medication doses night after night after night.

More boldly, what if we choose to draw the boundaries of the system more broadly or differently from the conventions? What if, as Duncan Neuhauser and his colleagues explore in Chapter Five, we draw the patient as existing *within* the system of his or her own care, instead of an *object* of the system of care? When we redraw boundaries, entirely new possibilities emerge.

Recent work by Wennberg[7] and by Kaplan and Greenfield[8,9] on active incorporation of patients into decision making is, in one view, centered directly on the systems issues of aims and on the differences between closed and open systems. A decision system formerly closed to involve only professionals maintains historical performance like a thermostat. Opening the system to outside influence, however, produces system outputs not characteristic of its own history. The open system seems to produce a better match between external needs and the output of the system. I am not sure that such jargon helps us understand the relevant health services research work because the jargon is not necessary. But what if we spring from this speculation to the larger and more pervasive question in the health care system as a whole: do we construct and maintain closed systems when we should value open ones?

The Sciences of Psychology in Systems

The second area of science in Deming's scheme he refers to as *psychology*. Four topics, at least, relate.

Sciences of Group Process. In many complex systems, interactions among people are crucial. Our work is done in exchanges—meetings, communications, markets, and groups of all sorts. How we interact in those groups is not a peripheral matter; it is central to the functioning of human systems. In understanding a system, it is not just the "boxes" (the elements) that count but also the "arrows" that connect the boxes (the dynamics among the elements). Our departments are different boxes; our meetings, our conversations, and our communications are the arrows.

Social and cognitive psychologists, anthropologists, economists, and others contribute to a store of knowledge about effective and ineffective group processes[10,11], yet those in most real work settings lack the skills and foresight to put this knowledge to use. Medical rounds, during which crucial decisions often are reached, follow the rituals of a past century, maintained as if nothing at all were known about better ways to work together. We reach allegedly scientific technical decisions with wholly unscientific group processes.

Sciences of Conflict Resolution. All systems experience internal and external friction. The heat that results is wasteful, and in human terms encourages suboptimization: local pride and competition thrive where cooperation would be better.

Economics, game theory, anthropology, linguistics, and sociobiology have each branched into understanding how conflicts arise and dissipate, how cooperation occurs, and, prescriptively, how the costs of friction can be minimized. By contrast, in the present medical care environment, our forms of handling disagreement remain primitive and uninformed by these sciences. With one important exception, we have yet to define cooperation building as a clinical skill. That exception is in our deepening understandings of how to improve the individual doctor-patient relationship, as represented in the work of Roter, Korsch, Inui, Stoeckle, and many others.[12]

Sciences of Understanding Motivation. Those in management systems have had a great deal of trouble breaking their addiction to primitive, mechanistic assumptions about motivation and incentive.

Very little evidence supports the pervasive use of reward, punishment, and contingent pay if what we want from our systems is continuous improvement.[13] A merit pay arrangement produces defensiveness, gaming, injured feelings, and suboptimization much more reliably than it produces better performance.

In place of outmoded ideas about rewards and punishments as a foundation for dealing with each other, we can substitute more modern evidence about the role of intrinsic motivators—pride, joy, affiliation, and celebration, for example—in human life.[14] Much more research remains to be done, but the issues for medical care are increasingly salient. As we doctors feel the pressure of increasing external control, we will have little more to rely on to maintain our joy in our work than deepening our understanding about where that joy comes from and how we can nurture and sustain it, lest both we and our patients suffer.

Creativity.   Perhaps most exciting among the areas of "scientific psychology" that can be applied are the modern efforts to understand creativity—the sources of new ideas that break through assumptions about closed systems. This is clearly a "softer" area of science than others, but a good deal is known about the characteristics of cultures, groups, organizations, and thought processes that promote or hinder creative development[15,16]. Charlie is a very talented singer; his ballads can bring tears to your eyes. Given the right opportunity and a few new skills, what might he invent that would help us all be better off? How very clever he is to hide the cards!

The Sciences of Learning, Prediction, and Experiment

The third domain in Deming's scheme is difficult to label, but I call it *the science of gaining knowledge*. Here, Deming draws from the works of John Dewey, C. I. Lewis[17], and others, asking as a formal matter how knowledge grows. It is a central matter for promoting improvement. Deming's scheme asked the question, By what methods do we learn?

However, there is an additional wrinkle. In many learning contexts, we seek to understand an existing universe. Our problem here, in Deming's terms, is "enumerative." We learn about the local distribution of mushrooms because we understand that such a local distribution exists. Perhaps we intend to take an action on this knowledge by picking them.

But what if we do not intend to *pick* mushrooms, but rather to plant them, so that we may harvest them in the future? The job of gaining knowledge is now different. There is no existing universe about which we can gain knowledge; we are not counting, we are "predicting." In characterizing the universe of existing mushrooms, there are boundaries to what we might want to know in order to make decisions: eight types of mushrooms, each in its own conceptual pot. But in deciding what to plant, the relevant questions are without bounds. The types of mushrooms may matter; so will the weather; so will the pests and rodents; so will the other planters of mushrooms; and so will the depth and spacing of planting. Even more, the harvest may be affected by factors about which we know nothing and by events that no one possibly can predict. We do not have a problem of enumeration, but instead a problem of prediction. We cannot know the truth because there is no truth yet to know.

How can we gain knowledge about a nonexistent future? This is the heart of the question that a doctor faces when treating an individual patient or that a manager faces when planning a task or project.

What forms of inquiry sustain the growth of knowledge in a dynamic, changing system? How can we be better predictors when we cannot know it all because "it all" hasn't happened yet?

Answers are neither certain nor crystal clear, but following the philosophers of epistemology, one plausible answer is this: Develop and maintain a system of cyclical, iterative investigation and learning that does its work in the real world and that keeps track of time as time passes. That is a bit complicated, so let's parse the concept.

First, our system of learning in a changing world must be cyclical because no collection of knowledge at any particular time can perfectly predict the future. We must be able to repeat the question because the answer may change. We must repeat the cycle often enough to follow the pace of change. What affects David's blood pressure tomorrow may differ substantially from what does so today.

Second, learning must be iterative, such that it builds on each new lesson and never assumes a fixed solution.

Third, we are interested not only in the process of investigation but also in the process of learning. Our method of gaining knowledge cannot be separated from the application of that knowledge. Therefore, it is important to ask *who* is gaining knowledge and whether and how that knowledge will be connected to action. John Dewey's view was that, at least among adults, "learning" is not separable from "action."[18]

Fourth, we are interested in the process of learning in a real world of action. This is not the same as relegating learning to a laboratory or to a specialized environment. Furthermore, this process is important not only in psychological terms, whereby adults learn through speaking and acting and not through passive listening, but also because prediction itself is grounded in the real world of local understanding. Growing mushrooms in Boston is similar to, but not quite the same as, growing mushrooms in Hanover, New Hampshire. The reason is very simple: things might happen that affect mushrooms grown in one place but not in the other. In fact, some things affect mushrooms in both places, but some things are local. To be as powerful as it can be, improvement must involve both local and general knowledge. In fact, the more we learn about improvement, the more powerful local factors seem to be.

Fifth and finally, our plan for gaining knowledge must have a sequential memory. It must keep accounts in temporal order. This order is necessary because the dimension of time is so closely interwoven with the task of prediction. A photograph of a golf ball in flight tells us very little about where it will land. A movie tells us a lot if we keep the frames in temporal order. In tasks of prediction, trajectories, histories, and trends can be highly informative.

Notice that histories and trends are not similarly informative in enumerative tasks. If I wish to pick them, I can pick mushrooms in any order I choose. However, in predicting how my mushrooms will grow, I may very much want to know how they have grown over time, day by day, and I also may want to know which way the temperature seems headed.

It is startling to me how little we apply the basic idea of preserving information over time to the care of our patients. We often summarize our patients' status as if we were photographing them in flight. We make lists, instead of graphs, and report trends far less formally than we report current status. In all of David's medical records, I found not a single graph of his blood pressures.

Walter Shewhart, the founding mind, if there was any, for what David Blumenthal calls the "industrial quality management sciences," asked why the process of scientific prediction could not be made part of the daily work of an organization.[19] He codified it as the "plan-do-check-act" cycle (PDCA), which is little more than shorthand for an experiment on the basis of which an action is to be taken. Alternatively, George Box calls this idea "the democratization of science." Box asserts that learning occurs when "capable observers" meet "informative events."[20] An experiment is the planned intersection of a capable observer with an informative event.

David's care is a series of potentially informative events within the visual field of potentially capable observers. The process of "experiment" that lies latent in his care, however, never matures into real, disciplined learning. As a result, predictions about the effects of actions taken remain uninformed—or insufficiently informed—by experience. At best, the decisions made are based far more on enumerative data ("in a series of one hundred patients with hypertension of renal origin, nifedipine produced . . .") than on analytical learning ("we systematically varied the dose of David's medication over a specific period, measured his blood pressure accurately and at appropriate times, and, on the basis of that trial, predict that his blood pressure will be controlled at the desired level under the followed regimen . . ."). Enumerative studies, correctly applied, often provide good hypotheses to test; analytical studies in the real world can help us make far better predictions.

For Charlie, the missed opportunity is to foster a trial of change in the system. Executives in high-performance organizations today embrace trials of change; "PDCA" is a way of life. Staff at most health care organizations do not embrace experiments in daily work. They give a hundred reasons why they cannot, and therefore the performance of the system remains as it has historically been— consistent with history.

The Sciences of Understanding Variation

The fourth area of science is *the science of variation*, or statistics.[21] Deming makes a strong case—perhaps too strong a case—that the statistics that should interest those of us attempting to improve real-world systems, the statistics that support prediction of the as-yet-unformed future, are quite different from the classical school-taught statistics focused on enumeration. In enumerative tasks, ideas such as significance testing and confidence intervals, for example, are quite meaningful. They measure, for example, the degree to which a sample may misrepresent the population. In prediction, however, these basic ideas of representativeness become fuzzy. How can one calculate the significance level of an estimate of a future that does not yet exist? Deming asserts there is no statistical theory for doing so.

Walter Shewhart actually used this difference to his advantage when he created the idea of the control chart.[19] Many a doctor has fretted over the idea that one can build a strong predictive model from a series of subgroup samples of three, two, or even one. For many, the "sample size" looks hopelessly small.

The answer is that Shewhart was not interested in describing a population based on a sample. He was interested in variation and stability over time and, for this purpose, extremely small samples were adequate as long as they were drawn rationally and contained ample time-dependent information. He was not as interested in asking, What has this machine produced? as he was in asking, Is this machine acting stably, or is it changing over time?

Control charts are one of the most powerful, practical tools ever developed in industry and can be used to inform interventions by both workers and managers. By recording efficiently and informatively the history of a process, a control chart could rapidly tell its user whether a specific new event is consistent with the past history of the process or the event was something unexpected and new. If the event is new, it is said to be "attributable" or of "special cause"; in such cases, investigating the event could be very informative. As Box describes it, "Someone spit in the batch."[20] If unexpected events are not observed over the history of the process, then the process or system is said to be "in control" and thereby evidences only "common causes" of variation.

The implications of this thinking for management were profound. Suppose a worker or a supervisor observed a random change due to variation inherent in the system but nonetheless treated it as special by investigating it or by asking for explanations or by adjusting the whole system in response. The result of such "tampering," as Deming describes it, was costly. It wasted time and energy (people "explained" why the coin came up heads *that* time), and it contributed to the variation of the system as a whole, similar to the way a child makes a swing go higher by pulling and pushing in phase with its initial oscillations.

Control charts helped people avoid tampering by using prescribed limits to guide interpretation of variation. Shewhart calls them "control limits" and suggests that they be set so as to limit the probability that people will act on random variation. Shewhart's "three-sigma" limits raise some debate in medical circles, where we are accustomed to enumerative rules involving significance levels of plus or minus *two* standard deviations, but we should not fuss too much about this. Shewhart's selection of three-sigma limits was a pragmatic and definitional decision. First, he observed a great deal of tampering in the real-world environments familiar to him, and he knew technically that a great deal more energy should be reserved instead for working on the common cause systems that set the limits on system performance. Second, he was not trying to discover whether causes were special or common. Instead, Shewhart was offering a *decision rule* on the basis of which action would either be taken or not. The three-sigma limit is a *definition*, not a *discovery*. For us, the policy question is, Which definition produces the wisest, most economical actions? rather than, Which definition most accurately classifies "truly" special and "truly" common causes?

No matter how we feel about the exact calculation of control limits, the notion of interpreting variation as a fundamental element in the science of improvement remains valid. The challenges are several: (1) to understand the basic concepts of special cause, common cause, and tampering; (2) to measure variables of importance in real-work settings as part of the work; (3) to display those measurements in the most informative possible formats, especially to help reduce tampering and to support PDCA cycles; and (4) to integrate all of these capabilities into the daily life of the organization, rather than leave them in the "research department."

In this volume, the reader will find many intriguing examples of how the processes of measurement and the interpretation of variation can be better integrated into the work of clinical care. These examples resonate strongly with the long history doctors already have of bringing better quantitative methods to clinical care. In the past few decades, doctors have learned to apply the methods of clinical epidemiology, decision theory, technology assessment, cost-effectiveness analysis, and more rigorous research design for clinical trials to understanding and improving medical care. In this context, incorporating the views of Shewhart and other industrial quality scientists into the work doctors do is a familiar task.

Conclusion

Armed with lessons from these improvement sciences—systems theory, psychology, experimentation in daily work, and understanding variation—I believe that we as doctors can become much more effective participants in the improvement of both patient care and the systems that house patient care. The scientific approaches, however, are not sufficient. To be effective, they must be applied within organizations and cultures capable of nurturing and sustaining them, much as scientific clinical work can thrive only in cultures where it is valued. To develop a culture of policy, behavior, and investment that will enable us to be scientists of improvement will not be easy. It will require substantial changes in our organizations and, indeed, in ourselves. But the power of these methods, in my mind, makes those changes well worth the effort. The choice we have as system leaders is quite clear. We can choose to remain trapped within systems that fail us, as were Charlie and David's helpers. Or, armed with sciences to inform our task, we can use knowledge to change and improve ineffective and inadequate systems to serve our shared and higher aims.

Notes

1. Nadler, G., & Hibino, S. (1990). *Breakthrough thinking*. Rocklin, CA: Prima.

2. Deming, W. E. (1993). *The new economics for industry, education, and government*. Cambridge: Massachusetts Institute of Technology, Center for Advanced Engineering Study.

3. Ackoff, R. L. (1984). *Creating the corporate future*. New York: Wiley.

4. Bertalanffy, L. (1968). *Genera: Systems theory: Foundation, development, applications*. New York: Braziller.

5. Senge, P. M. (1990). *The fifth discipline: The art and practice of the learning organization*. New York: Doubleday.

6. Ackoff, R. L. (1984). *Creating the corporate future*. New York: Wiley, p. 99.

7. Wennberg, J. E. (1988). Improving the decision-making process. *Health Affairs, 7*, 99–106.

8. Greenfield, S., Kaplan, S. H., & Ware, J. E., Jr. (1985). Expanding

patient involvement in care: Effects on patient outcomes. *Annals of Internal Medicine, 102,* 520–528.

9. Kaplan, S. H., Greenfield, S., & Ware, J. E., Jr. (1989). Assessing the effects of physician-patient interactions on the outcomes of chronic disease. *Medical Care, 27*(Suppl.), S110–S127.

10. Sholtes, P. R. (1988). *The team handbook.* Madison, WI: Joiner Associates.

11. Katzenbach, J. R., & Smith, D. K. (1993). *The wisdom of teams: Creating the high-performance organization.* Boston: Harvard Business School Press.

12. Stewart, M., & Roter, D. L. (Eds.). (1989). *Communicating with patients in medical practice.* Newbury Park, CA: Sage.

13. Herzberg, F. M. (1968). One more time: How do you motivate employees? *Harvard Business Review, 65,* 109–120.

14. Condry, J., & Chambers, J. (1981). Intrinsic motivation and the process of learning. In W. A. Collins (Ed.), *Aspects of the development of competence: The Minnesota Symposium on Child Psychology* (Vol. 14, pp. 61–84). Hillsdale, NJ: Erlbaum.

15. de Bono, E. (1992). *Serious creativity.* New York: HarperCollins.

16. Fritz, R. (1991). *Creating.* New York: Fawcett.

17. Lewis, C. I. (1929). *Mind and the world order.* New York: Scribner.

18. Senge, P. M. (1990). The leader's new work: Building learning organizations. *Sloan Management Review, 32,* 7–23.

19. Shewhart, W. (1980). *Economic control of quality of manufactured product.* Milwaukee: ASQC Quality Press. (Original work published 1931)

20. Box, G. (1993). Personal testimony.

21. Wheeler, D. J. (1993). *Understanding variation: The key to managing chaos.* Knoxville, TN: SPC Press.

2

Applying Industrial Quality Management Science to Physicians' Clinical Decisions

David Blumenthal, M.D., M.P.P.

Increasing concerns with the quality of health care have led to experimentation with and deployment of multiple new technologies designed to monitor, compare, and improve the clinical performance of health care providers.[1] Among the newest and most controversial of these approaches is industrial quality management science (IQMS), also known as continuous quality improvement (CQI), the quality improvement process (QIP), and total quality management (TQM).[2,3,4]

Evidence of the rapid spread of IQMS as an approach to managing quality in health care institutions is widespread. The Joint Commission for the Accreditation of Health Care Organizations has adopted IQMS as an important standard in its reviews of health care institutions.[5] On the basis of a recent national survey, editors at *Hospitals* magazine estimate that 3,100 U.S. hospitals with more than fifty beds now have programs in TQM.[6] "If you don't already have Total Quality Management (TQM) fever," *Hospitals* editors

The author gratefully acknowledges the very helpful comments and suggestions of Drs. Donald Berwick, Paul Plsek, and Steven Skates in the preparation of the manuscript for this chapter.

tell their readership, "chances are you'll catch it soon."[6] In Massachusetts a recent revision of the state's hospital financing law included a section establishing a commission "to collect and disseminate evidence for the value and success of recognized quality improvement principles and methods . . . including but not limited to Total Quality Management" (Section 59, Chapter 495 of the General Laws of the Commonwealth of Massachusetts).

Despite the apparent popularity of IQMS among health care managers, however, many physicians have reacted with skepticism.[2,4,7] One explanation for this resistance may be the failure of proponents of IQMS to develop and communicate a convincing theoretical, empirical, and practical case that the techniques and activities of IQMS are applicable to the primary work that clinicians do—namely, the management of individual patients' medical problems. In this chapter, I explore at a conceptual level the potential applicability of certain facets of IQMS to physicians' clinical decisions.

IQMS: Basic Principles

The basic tenets of IQMS have been well described elsewhere.[2-4,7-10] For now it is enough to note that three activities generally are emphasized as central to this approach to quality management. These are, in Berwick's[11] words:

1. Efforts to know the customer ever more deeply and to link that knowledge ever more closely to the day-to-day activities of the organization;
2. Efforts to mold the culture of the organization, largely through deeds of leaders, to foster pride, joy, collaboration, and scientific thinking;
3. Efforts to continuously increase knowledge of and control over variation in the processes of work through the widespread use of scientific methods of collection, analysis and action upon data.

Many of the specific tools and techniques that have become emblematic of IQMS were developed to support the third of these three elements. These tools offer quick and efficient methods for displaying and analyzing data.[9]

The enthusiasm for this doctrine and set of analytical tools stems partly from their apparent effectiveness in other countries and industries, especially Japan.[12-14] In health care, interest in IQMS also has spread because certain aspects of the work of health care organizations (for example, the support and hotel functions of hospitals) are so similar to other industries that IQMS seems readily applicable to these functional areas.[3] Furthermore, an increasing anecdotal literature describes the success of IQMS in analyzing, ameliorating, and solving particular health care problems.[3,15-19] For example, a recent report credits IQMS with reducing the rate of postoperative wound infections from 1.8 percent to 0.4 percent at Intermountain Health Care's LDS Hospital in Salt Lake City.[20,21]

Encouraging as these accounts are, however, doubts linger in the minds of some health care observers about the long-term value of this new philosophy of quality management. Even enthusiasts of IQMS note that they have never encountered a sector quite like health care. A principal reason is the role of the physician. Robert King, executive director of Goal/QPC, a well-respected Massachusetts consulting group that specializes in IQMS, noted in a recent interview: "I think that the fact that in most hospitals most physicians are not employees and are fairly autonomous is quite a different . . . situation from a manufacturing organization . . . I think we need to do a lot more work figuring out how to deal with the situation where you have all of these non-employees who play such a critical role in the organization."[18]

The autonomy of physicians and their central role in resource allocation within the health care system generally makes their active participation in and support of new quality improvement initiatives vital to these programs' success. As Berwick[11] and others have noted, however, physicians have proven resistant to IQMS. The sources of this resistance seem to include:

1. Physicians' general resistance to change,[22] an attribute they share with many other professional and nonprofessional groups

2. Their fear that IQMS's emphasis on reducing variation in the process of care will lead to an attack on their autonomy, their ability to vary care to meet the needs of particular patients, and their ability to innovate[11]

3. The fact that early applications of IQMS have been championed by administrators and have been used primarily to address problems perceived as the responsibility of administration[7]; physicians are frequently distrustful of administrators in health care organizations[22]

4. The strong emphasis of IQMS on breaking down professional boundaries and developing interdisciplinary teams, which many physicians find threatening to their status in health care organizations[4,23]

These issues alone would constitute important obstacles to the involvement of physicians in IQMS, but one difficulty remains that could prove as important as any of the others. *Advocates of IQMS are only beginning to develop, and have not yet refined, a persuasive theoretical, empirical, and practical argument that the techniques and activities of IQMS can improve the decisions that individual physicians make for their patients.*

Although not sufficient, the elaboration of such a case is almost certainly necessary to the long-term success of IQMS among physicians. Physicians seem unlikely to involve themselves wholeheartedly in IQMS until they understand how its methods and approaches are relevant to the work they view as their own. This attitude does not necessarily reflect either self-centeredness or disinterest in self-improvement. Even the most flexible and broadminded clinicians must set priorities concerning where to invest their scarce time in attempting to better their own performance.

The conscientious practitioner today is awash in new knowledge concerning medical practices and procedures that may have direct bearing on his or her patients' health and welfare and that no other health professional has the skills or legal authority to employ. The literature also is replete with studies and commentaries demonstrating how slow practicing physicians are to digest and respond to this new information.[22,24-27] Under these circumstances, a tendency for physicians to concentrate their efforts at self-improvement in areas that seem most pertinent to their patient care responsibilities would seem natural and predictable.

Furthermore, a very promising time to educate physicians concerning the principles and practices of IQMS is during medical school and residency.[28] Currently, these educational experiences emphasize case-by-case encounters with patients in which learning and improving the process of clinical decision making is the critical task. Until medical education is significantly changed or until IQMS proves its relevance to the current approach, IQMS may remain tangential to what most physicians (rightly or wrongly) perceive as their role.

Potential Applicability of IQMS to Clinical Decision Making

Why should we think that IQMS and its techniques might be useful to clinicians in their management of patients? Although definitive evidence remains to be developed, the conceptual and scientific underpinnings of IQMS have important similarities to tools that increasingly are advocated and used by scholars and practitioners in the fields of decision analysis, clinical epidemiology, outcomes research, and effectiveness research. Furthermore, it is possible to imagine circumstances in which IQMS might be extremely useful to patient management in day-to-day clinical situations. To understand these areas of potential applicability, a very brief digression into the history and techniques of IQMS is useful.

Evolution of Industrial Quality Management Science (IQMS)

Industrial quality management science (IQMS) began in the early twentieth century as an effort to use elementary principles of statistics to measure variation in the processes of production, to identify sources of that variation, to reduce it, and thereby to ensure the quality of resulting products. The emphasis was on control: controlling manufacturing processes so as to control (maintain) the level of quality. Eventually, however, the techniques used for controlling quality were applied also to its improvement.

Perhaps the most widely known and important tool to emerge from this early phase of IQMS is Shewhart's control chart.[11,12] A simplified example of this device is illustrated in Figure 2.1. The vertical axis measures some aspect of a process or product that is considered vital from a quality standpoint. The horizontal axis measures time. The solid line represents the mean of the observed values. The dashed lines represent upper and lower control limits, which generally are set at two or three standard deviations above or below the mean. Typically, control limits indicate the amount of variation expected in a process that is considered "in control" or "stable." The decision concerning where to place such boundaries is discretionary (for example, at two versus three standard deviations from the mean). This decision should take into account the comparative costs of concluding that a process is stable when it is unstable, or unstable when it is not. Wider limits will predispose to the first type of error (Type I) and narrower limits to the second type (Type II).

The control chart allows rapid and accurate assessment of the significance of observed variation in a process of production. Such variation is endemic in all systems. Control charts also provide information about whether such variations reflect random factors (for example, minor discrepancies in the performance of machines, personnel, or characteristics of raw materials) or whether they derive from a change in underlying performance of the process

FIGURE 2.1 Typical Control Chart

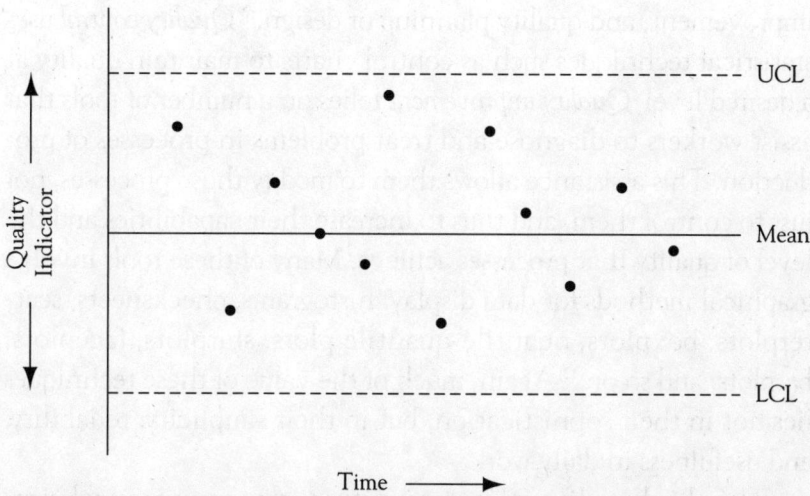

Note: UCL = Upper control limit; LCL = Lower control limit.
Source: Blumenthal, D. (1993). Total quality management and physicians' clinical decisions. *Journal of the American Medical Association*, 269(21), 2775–2778. Copyright © 1993, American Medical Association. Reprinted by permission.

under observation. Such a change would be signaled when quality measures fall outside the control limits, thus indicating that the process is no longer functioning predictably at its former level. This occurrence may require a response to protect the quality of the product.

The value of the control chart lies not in the novelty of the statistical principles underlying it, but *in the ease and reliability with which it converts data into information*. In the words of Wadsworth, Stephens, and Godfrey,[12] control charts are "*analytical visualizations* [italics added] of the corresponding distribution of the computed statistics on quality characteristics being studied." The application of the control chart and other related techniques is generally known as *statistical quality control* (SQC). Much of the intellectual work undergirding SQC was accomplished before and during World War II.[12,29]

The techniques of SQC can be used to advance the quality of products through three types of activities: quality control, quality improvement, and quality planning or design.[12] *Quality control* uses statistical techniques such as control charts to maintain quality at a desired level. *Quality improvement* relies on a number of tools that assist workers to diagnose and treat problems in processes of production. This assistance allows them to modify those processes, not just to control them, and thus to increase their capabilities and the level of quality that processes achieve. Many of these tools involve graphical methods for data display: histograms, checksheets, scatterplots, boxplots, quantile-quantile plots, starplots, faceplots, barplots, and so on.[12] Again, much of the value of these techniques lies not in their sophistication, but in their simplicity, reliability, and usefulness in daily work.

The third quality-related activity, *quality planning or design*, involves techniques whose purpose is to "design-in quality" by developing products that are both superior in quality (for example, capability, reliability, durability, appearance) and easier to manufacture. Among these techniques are methods for assessing preferences of consumers and for incorporating those preferences into the designs of products and of processes for producing them. In the automobile industry and other settings, such approaches have been used to greatly reduce the time it takes to design a new product and to make such products more responsive to the wishes of ultimate consumers.

To understand the differences between quality control, quality improvement, and quality design, imagine a process for performing CT scans of the human brain. Quality control activities would attempt to ensure that the resolution of these CT scans is the best that a given machine can achieve on every imaging attempt. Quality improvement activities might seek ways to improve significantly the resolution the machine can attain, perhaps through modifications in its software or hardware. Quality design activities might result in a rethinking of the CT scan as an imaging device and the consequent development of an entirely new imaging technology with qualitatively superior capabilities, such as magnetic resonance imaging.

Distinctions among these three quality-related activities are not absolute. Efforts to control quality by documenting variation, analyzing its sources, and reducing it may lead to improvements in the capabilities of machines and even may inspire changes in design. At a conceptual level, however, it is useful to distinguish these three components of quality management.

A second phase in the evolution of IQMS began in the 1950s with the introduction of the concept of total quality control (TQC).[30] Prior to this time, the techniques of SQC had been used increasingly in industry, but they were applied for the most part by special departments with responsibility for the management of quality. All too frequently, such quality departments did not detect problems until they had been present for some time. Also, personnel in other units in the organization often resisted the advice of quality managers. The solution, according to Feigenbaum and others, was to decentralize the management of quality and the use of statistical quality techniques. All units and divisions of a company should have engineers or specialized personnel with the capability of using SQC. The result, it was hoped, would be prompter attention to quality problems and greater acceptance of solutions. Thus, by the early post–World War II period, the evolution of IQMS had shifted from a focus on the development of new statistical techniques to a concentration on reforms in management that would ensure the use of SQC.

A third phase in the evolution of IQMS was pioneered by the Japanese in the mid-1970s. They developed the concept of companywide quality control (CWQC), the purpose of which is to involve all employees of an organization in the activities of quality control, quality improvement, and quality planning, and thereby to ensure that these techniques achieve their full potential. CWQC also places a premium on personal leadership by senior management in the effort to improve quality, on making the improvement of quality an essential element in the strategy of an organization, and on changing organizational values and culture so that quality is elevated above profit making as a goal.

An important figure in the development of the theory and

practice of CWQC was W. Edwards Deming, a physicist and statistician who had spent much of his life perfecting the techniques of SQC. Deming had been deeply disappointed by the failure of post–World War II American industry to implement SQC or TQC. During the war, many American manufacturing organizations had adopted the techniques of SQC because the U.S. military insisted on them. Immediately after the war, however, most American companies discarded SQC because senior management regarded it as a government imposition and never learned or supported it. As Deming[8] notes: "the flare of statistical methods by themselves, in an atmosphere in which management did not know their responsibilities, burned, sputtered, fizzled and died out . . . It was vital not to repeat in Japan," he writes, " the mistakes made in America."

CWQC is the approach to quality management that many leading non-health-care companies (for example, Xerox, Ford Motor Company, Hewlett-Packard, Motorola) currently employ. When health care reformers now refer to IQMS (or CQI, QIP, or TQM), it is generally this last stage in the development of industrial quality methods that they would like to see adopted in health care organizations. Figure 2.2 provides a schematic summary of the evolution of IQMS.

In some industrial organizations that have adopted modern quality methods, approaches to quality have evolved over time from SQC to TQC to CWQC, thus repeating the learning process that the field as a whole went through during the course of the twentieth century. A few companies have jumped directly to implementing CWQC. In the health care system at the current time, leaders and managers frequently are urged to adopt the concepts of CWQC immediately, without first experimenting with SQC and TQC.

One of the reasons that physicians have lagged behind in recent efforts to introduce modern quality methods may be their discomfort with leaping immediately to a stage in quality management that emphasizes managerial and administrative changes, such as reforms in organizational "culture," topics with which physicians have trouble identifying. It is not uncommon, for example, to hear of physi-

FIGURE 2.2 Evolution of Industrial Quality Management Science (IQMS)

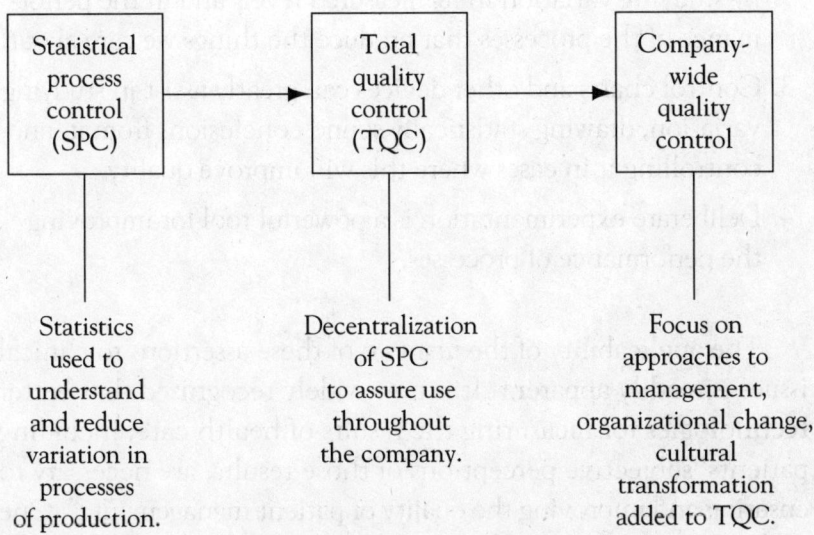

| Statistical process control (SPC) | → | Total quality control (TQC) | → | Company-wide quality control |
| Statistics used to understand and reduce variation in processes of production. | | Decentralization of SPC to assure use throughout the company. | | Focus on approaches to management, organizational change, cultural transformation added to TQC. |

cians who have been turned into skeptics because a brief, initial encounter with the ideas of IQMS emphasized such (to them) foreign notions as empowerment of workers, fostering joy and collaboration in the workplace, and breaking down departmental boundaries.

The managerial components of industrial quality methods have been crucial to their success in industry and may prove in the end to be their most important contribution to performance in health care organizations. For the work of individual physicians, however, the applicability of SQC, a set of tools developed at earlier stages in the evolution of what is now called IQMS, is more immediately and intuitively apparent.

Statistical Quality Control and Clinical Care

Among the many insights into quality control and improvement embodied in SQC are the following:

1. Quality must be measured to be controlled or improved.

2. Much can be learned about how to control or improve quality by studying variation in its measured levels and in the performance of the processes that produce the things we care about.

3. Control charts and other devices can greatly assist in studying variation, drawing statistically sound conclusions from it, and controlling it in cases where this will improve quality.

4. Deliberate experimentation is a powerful tool for improving the performance of processes.

The applicability of the first two of these assertions to clinical issues is readily apparent. It is now widely recognized that better technologies for measuring the results of health care, including patients' subjective perceptions of those results, are necessary to ensuring and improving the quality of patient management.[1,31] One of the principal activities of the diverse field now called "outcomes research" has been the development, validation, and application of such measures.[32] The Medical Outcomes Study, for example, has had as a central purpose the development of "practical tools for monitoring patient outcomes and their determinants in routine practice."[1,33] The federal government's recent creation of patient outcomes research teams (PORTs) and the Medical Effectiveness Program are further evidence of the increasing consensus on the need for better and more practical measures of quality that can be applied to the evaluation and improvement of everyday patient services.[34]

The second insight of SQC, the importance of studying variation in process and outcomes, is also increasingly applied in clinical care. Much of the current concern with health care quality has its origin in this very phenomenon of variation: in this case, the documentation of unexplained variation in the processes and outcomes of care across institutions and geographical locales.[11,32,35] Having used observed variation in clinical practice as a cudgel to get the attention of policymakers and professionals, scholars now are trying to draw information from analysis of variation so as to improve the processes of care and thus their outcomes. This is a central goal of clinical epidemiology, which uses statistical tools of inference like those of SQC to test hypotheses about the relationships between process and outcomes in clinical services. Indeed, leading clinical journals commonly contain articles that analyze the processes of care or service using epidemiological techniques and constructs with which Shewhart, Feigenbaum, Juran, Deming, and other industrial quality experts would be completely comfortable and which they began applying to industrial problems before World War II.

Not surprisingly, the Department of Clinical Epidemiology at Intermountain Health Care did the work referred to above that led to the reduction in postoperative wound infections at that hospital.[20] Staff started by describing variation in the rates of wound infection among patients of different physicians and showed that the timing of administration of prophylactic antibiotics explained a good deal of that variation. They further showed that patients who received their antibiotics two hours before surgery had the lowest infection rates.[19] The Surgery Department adopted a policy that all patients should receive prophylaxis precisely two hours before their operations, and the fall in infection rates followed.

The techniques of SQC may hold special promise for improving the delivery of primary care. Most primary care involves patients who are either basically healthy or chronically ill. The goal is to maintain health or to prevent it from deteriorating further. In either case, patients' health status is stable for long periods of time, and the physician endeavors to keep it that way (or to improve it, if he or she knows how).

In this circumstance, one can view the processes of normal and abnormal physiology as being "in control" or stable, just as an industrial process might be. Indeed, the human organism depends in both sickness and health on a vast system of physiological processes that are exquisitely controlled through a variety of mechanisms. The outputs of such processes commonly are measured parameters such

as weight, heart rate, blood pressure, temperature, serum cholesterol, serum glucose, hematocrit, prothrombin time, and arterial
oxygen saturation. Regulation occurs through such diverse mechanisms as the pituitary-adrenal axis, sympathetic and parasympathetic pathways, hemostasis and the clotting cascade, baroreceptors
in carotid sinus and aortic arch, the renin-angiotensin system, and
a legion of other biochemical, neuronal, and hydraulic devices. One
challenge facing the primary care physician is to measure, interpret,
and react appropriately to variations in these "stable" processes. For
example, primary practitioners must deal with such questions as
how often to measure blood pressure in hypertensive individuals or
prothrombin times in anticoagulated patients, how to interpret
changes in such parameters over time, and how to judge whether
those changes justify any action on the part of physician or patient.

These are precisely the types of problems that SQC has been
used to address with respect to stable industrial processes. One sus-
pects that the experienced physician uses the equivalent of a control chart all the time by mentally posing the question: is this blood
pressure (or weight, or prothrombin level, or serum glucose, or peak
flow rate) significantly different from previous measures? Do I need
to do something about this value? The answer generally is inferred
from rapid review of the old record. Physicians undoubtedly vary in
their ability to make such informal assessments. Even if the experienced physician generally reaches the appropriate answer, the
process of instructing medical students and residents on how to
interpret flows of data concerning patient health status could be
greatly assisted by the use of SQC.

Figure 2.3 shows how a control chart might be applied in monitoring an anticoagulated patient's monthly prothrombin ratio during one year. In this case, the observed mean over the period under
review has been 16.1 seconds. The upper and lower control limits
represent two standard deviations from the mean of the patient's
observed prothrombin ratio over the previous twelve months.

The control chart displays the patient's laboratory data in a
readily consumable form. It allows rapid and statistically sound
appraisal of whether the desired level of hemostasis has been

FIGURE 2.3 Monthly Recordings of Prothrombin Ratios (Patient/Control) in Anticoagulated Patient with Mechanical Heart Valve

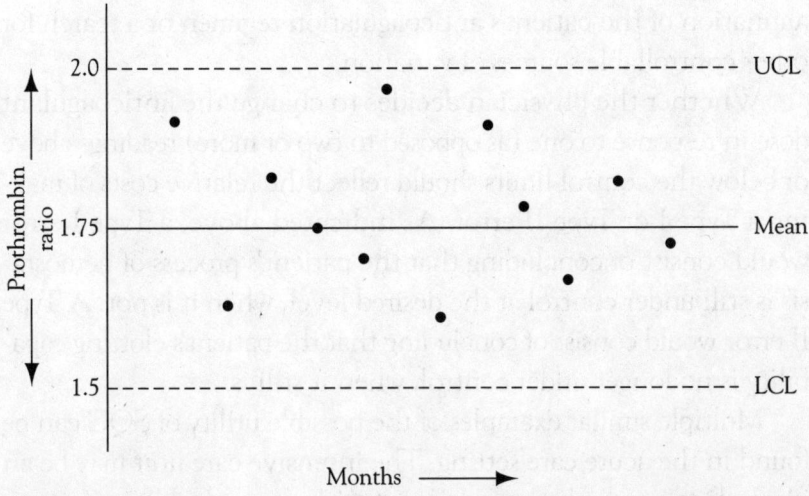

Note: UCL = Upper control limit = 2.0; LCL = Lower control limit = 1.5
Source: Blumenthal, D. (1993). Total quality management and physicians' clinical decisions. *Journal of the American Medical Association*, 269(21), 2775–2778. Copyright © 1993, American Medical Association. Reprinted by permission.

reached (the mean PTR) and of the stability of that level (apparent both in the control limits and in the variability of observed PTRs over time). Once such a pattern has been established, control charts also help clinicians interpret the significance of future values. For the patient in Figure 2.3, statistical principles tell us that if the underlying physiology of hemostasis is unchanged and if the dose of anticoagulant is constant, then the PTR will be above the upper control limit by chance only 5 times in 100 measurements. Two consecutive PTRs will be greater than two standard deviations above the mean only 2.5 times in 1,000 by chance alone, and three consecutive PTRs will be above the upper control limit only 1.2 times in 10,000 by chance (assuming that values are normally distributed and independent of one another). The occurrence of these values or patterns could indicate that the patient's underlying process of hemostasis is no longer "in control" at the desired level. For some physicians or some patients (for example, those at greater than average risk of bleeding), this possibility may justify a reexamination of the patient's anticoagulation regimen or a search for other controllable sources of variation.

Whether the physician decides to change the anticoagulant dose in response to one (as opposed to two or more) readings above or below the control limits should reflect the relative costs of making a Type I or Type II error. As indicated above, a Type I error would consist of concluding that the patient's process of hemostasis is still under control at the desired level, when it is not. A Type II error would consist of concluding that the patient's clotting capability is no longer under control, when it still is.

Multiple similar examples of the possible utility of SQC can be found in the acute care setting. The intensive care unit may be an ideal place in which to experiment with the techniques of statistical process control. The complexity of the process of care and the multiple personnel involved create opportunity for confusion, miscommunication, and delay. Variations in key parameters must be interpreted by multiple different actors on the same team and on different teams of providers. What does a transient dip in arterial oxygen saturation mean to the nurse responsible for pulmonary toilet, compared with the anesthesiologist who is ICU attending or the respiratory technician who adjusts the ventilator? Different team members display data in different ways within and among intensive care units in the same institution. This greatly complicates and delays the work of consultants who must go from unit to unit, providing advice on particular organ systems or problems. The talented and experienced consultant may overcome inconsistencies to reach appropriate inferences most of the time. But what about the average clinician or the clinician who is tired or rushed? Once again, SQC was developed to increase understanding of complex processes that yield a stream of data over time and to help personnel managing those processes to react consistently and appropriately.

An equally interesting possibility is that aspects of SQC could be taught by physicians or nurses to their patients so that the patients could make more intelligent decisions about the management of their own health. Imagine, for example, the following approach to involving patients in the care of their own systolic hypertension. As part of routine management, patients are instructed in how to keep a control chart and are asked to take their blood pressure on a regular basis (perhaps weekly) and to record the results. Figure 2.4 illustrates what such a control chart might look like for a patient with systolic hypertension whose pressure has been brought "under control" through the use of medications. For each such patient, the physician could establish a rule concerning how much variability is acceptable and instruct the patient in how to respond if the rule is violated. For example, one patient with near critical carotid artery stenosis is instructed to call if one reading drops below the 130 line or if more than three consecutive readings are below the mean. Another patient with no risk factors for end-organ complications is told that he should call if two out of three consecutive readings are above or below the control limits or if four readings in a row are above or below the mean.

This approach would have several advantages. It could reduce the number of visits to doctors' offices by hypertensives and thus reduce the costs of primary care. The approach would result also in earlier detection of loss of control and thus decrease the amounts of time that patients would be out of control over a lifetime of anti-hypertensive treatment. The routine monitoring of blood pressure by patients also makes it possible to investigate such questions as the magnitude and significance of variability of blood pressure in the "controlled" hypertensive over long periods of time. How much effort should physicians be exerting to keep blood pressure within one or two standard deviations of the desired mean? This issue has received considerable attention in the diabetic population. The use of control charts would facilitate its exploration in this patient group, as well.

An objection might be that use of control charts requires

FIGURE 2.4 Systolic Blood Pressure Before and After Treatment

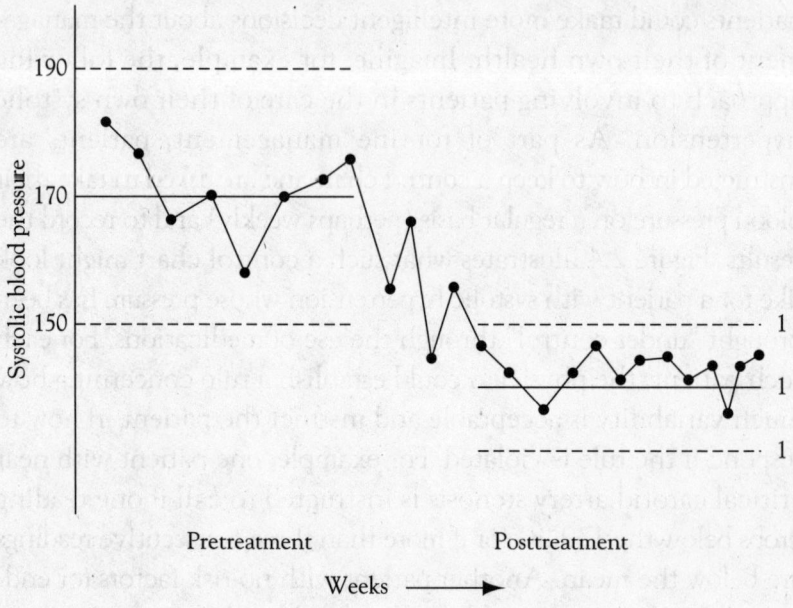

patients to take a great deal of responsibility for participating in their own care. Clearly, not every patient would be willing or able to play this role. But if assembly line workers can use SQC to enhance Toyota's or Honda's profits, they should be equally capable of using those techniques (and far more motivated) in interpreting measurements of their own blood pressure, blood sugar, cholesterol, or weight.

Other, more sophisticated applications of SQC have potential applicability to improving clinical decision making. Particularly interesting are tools for quality improvement and quality design used in industrial settings. Over the years, practitioners of IQMS have developed sophisticated techniques to improve quality through, among other things, organizing, conducting, and learning from experiments with industrial processes.[12]

Here again, certain obvious parallels to clinical care become apparent. Experimentation is the linchpin of progress in clinical decision making. In that sense, professionals in the clinical sciences long ago discovered and implemented this approach to quality improvement.

The contribution of IQMS in this area may be found in its development of simplified techniques for conducting valid experiments during the course of daily operations.[12] A problem with traditional experimental approaches in clinical sciences is their cost and the difficulty of organizing them. This problem has led to their isolation from the mainstream of practice and to resulting problems in translating results into clinical care. Furthermore, it is widely recognized that clinicians experiment every day with patient management but may not currently have the tools to learn from such experiments.[32]

SQC may offer some help with these problems in applying experimental methods to learning about patient care. Take, for example, evolutionary operations (EVOP), a technique developed in the 1950s by G.E.P. Box, a statistician and a scholar of industrial organization and quality management.[12] The purpose of EVOP is to assist in the evolutionary improvement of processes by continually conducting small, nondisruptive but statistically meaningful experiments. The technique is similar to nonrandomized clinical experimentation but is simplified for application by unsophisticated personnel. It allows and encourages personnel to vary sequentially the various factors that they think may affect an important outcome and to observe the effects and make inferences from those effects.

Could EVOP or similar techniques be applied to the daily work of a clinician or of a clinical unit? In principle, a motivated primary care physician or group could periodically vary one aspect of the way they manage certain diseases or approaches to patient care (holding other aspects constant) and measure the results. Indeed, this already may take place much more commonly than we appreciate. The major obstacles may be precisely in the details: finding ways to conduct such mini-experiments inexpensively, efficiently, and nondisruptively; accumulating enough trials (a large enough sample) to draw statistically valid conclusions; and devising systems in advance to learn from the results.

Computer technology offers new opportunities to accomplish these tasks, both in industry and in health care, by connecting isolated practitioners to networks that will pool their experiences and generate feedback in real time. More sophisticated approaches to outcomes research, such as those envisioned by Mulley,[32] seem similar to EVOP. EVOP probably would prove most readily applicable to situations that occur frequently in a clinician's experience—for example, in uncomplicated elective surgery or in management of uncomplicated hypercholesterolemia. If techniques of SQC can facilitate this process, then teaching these techniques to physicians-in-training could give them powerful tools for lifetime learning. Teaching SQC and other aspects of IQMS to practicing physicians could measurably augment the quality of care they provide.

Another technique that has been long used in IQMS and that is now increasingly applied to quality management in health care is flowcharting. Flowcharts break complex processes into sequences of steps. This division allows the identification of unnecessary or poorly designed aspects of a process and facilitates its modification. In health care, flowcharts have long been used for teaching purposes. Every new intern now carries around manuals that provide very clear instructions on how to care for common clinical situations. In the guise of guidelines and "critical paths," flowcharts also are used increasingly by professional societies and health care organizations as educational devices for practicing physicians. Flowcharts have additional potential, however, as analytical devices for understanding the sources of variability in the care of patients and opportunities for improving what physicians do in their daily practice. Here the emphasis is on describing as precisely as possible what a physician actually does with and for his or her patients, rather than on what ought to be done. The current process then becomes the substrate upon which improvement can be built.

Inconsistencies Between IQMS and Physician Decision Making

Similarities between the problems that physicians confront and that IQMS is designed to approach should not obscure the contrasts. One of the central issues facing clinicians and industrial decision makers is the need to make decisions in the face of uncertainty. In the physician's case, there is uncertainty about the causes of presenting symptoms and signs, about the effectiveness and side effects of alternative treatments, about the natural history of disease in particular circumstances, and about the psychological, social, and economic circumstances of patients. In the case of industry, there may be uncertainty about the quality of raw materials, about the reliability of machinery, about the training of workers, and about how a complex system of processes interacts to create quality problems.

In both clinical and industrial settings, such uncertainties can be reduced through the diligent collection and display of data, from the application of appropriate tools of statistical inference and through the use of scientific methods for diagnosing and ameliorating the causes of pathological processes. The goal in both settings is to use past experience to make the results of future work more predictable: the work of maintaining health, diagnosing and treating illness, manufacturing a product, or serving a customer.

Physicians, however, face limits on their ability to reduce uncertainty that do not affect industrial workers. One irreducible source of uncertainty for physicians is the individuality of each human being and the potential uniqueness of his or her problems, needs, and responses. This potential uniqueness limits the physician's ability to use experience with past patients to predict how future patients will respond to interventions. The difficulty is particularly great in situations in which patients combine multiple complex problems. A common example is the diabetic patient on multiple medications who suffers from heart disease, renal disease, and hypertension and then presents with new onset of dizziness.

But lack of predictability is inherent in every patient encounter and cannot be eliminated. Even in so-called uncomplicated hypertension, responses to medications are unpredictable. Industrial processes can be complex and unpredictable as well, but at least they can be run over and over so that their variability can be characterized. The same patient cannot be subjected (for both ethical and practical reasons) again and again to the same surgical procedure or to the initiation of the same medication.

A second reason why physicians deal with greater uncertainty than industry managers and workers pertains to the complexity of biological processes and the limits on doctors' ability to learn about them. Although industrial processes may be complex, few rival the human organism (or any living being) in the number and diversity of processes that are operating simultaneously to produce outcomes of interest. Furthermore, no matter how complex an industrial process, it theoretically can be stopped, disassembled, studied, and reassembled. To be sure, there will be a cost, but at least the opportunity exists. The same cannot be said under any circumstances for the biological processes with which physicians must deal.

These considerations suggest that IQMS may not be applicable equally to all of the important clinical situations that physicians face and that its potential in this regard should not be overstated. Beyond this, the ultimate test of the utility of IQMS in clinical problem solving will consist of empirical evidence of its ability to improve the processes and outcomes of care. Such evidence undoubtedly will take considerable time to develop.

The need for caution in addressing such issues, however, should not obscure the importance of doing so. As clinical care grows more complex, physicians in daily practice need to be equipped with tools that will enable them and their patients to turn data into information as quickly and efficiently as possible. IQMS offers potentially valuable devices for accomplishing this task and for empowering physicians to improve continually their management of patients. In the process, physicians may come to understand also whether

IQMS will prove just the latest fad in health care management or whether it has the potential for making health care organizations into powerful engines for meeting the needs and expectations of the individuals they serve.

Notes

1. Greenfield, S., & Nelson, E. C. (1992). Recent developments and future issues in the use of health status assessment measures in clinical settings. *Medical Care, 30*(Suppl. 5), 1–19.

2. Berwick, D. M. (1989). Continuous improvement as an ideal in health care. *New England Journal of Medicine, 320,* 53–56.

3. Laffel, G., & Blumenthal, D. (1989). The case for using industrial quality management science in health care organizations. *Journal of the American Medical Association, 262,* 2869–2873.

4. Berwick, D. M., Enthoven, A., & Bunker, J. P. (1992). Quality management in the NHS: The doctor's role. *British Medical Journal, 304,* 235–239, 304–308.

5. O'Leary, D. S. (1992). Agenda for change fosters CQI concepts. *Joint Commission Perspectives,* (January/February), 2–3.

6. Grayson, M. A. (1992). Benchmark TQM survey tracks a new management era in administration. 66(11), 26–27.

7. Berwick, D. M., Godfrey, A. B., & Roessner, J. (1990). *Curing health care: New strategies for quality improvement.* San Francisco: Jossey-Bass.

8. Deming, W. E. (1986). *Out of the crisis.* Cambridge: MIT-CAES. (p. 26)

9. Scherkenbach, W. B. (1986). *The Deming route.* Washington, DC: CEEP Press.

10. Juran, J. M. (1989). *Juran on leadership for quality: An executive handbook.* New York: Free Press.

11. Berwick, D. M. (1991). Controlling variation in health care: A consultation from Walter Shewhart. *Medical Care, 29*(12), 1212–1225.

12. Wadsworth, H. M., Stephens, K. S., & Godfrey, A. B. (1986). *Modern methods for quality control and improvement.* New York: Wiley. (p. 121)

13. Walton, M. (1986). *The Deming management method.* New York: Putnam.

14. Garvin, D. A. (1988). *Managing quality: The strategic and competitive edge.* New York: Free Press.

15. Kuperman, G., James, B., Jacobsen, J., & Gardner, R. M. (1991). Continuous quality improvement applied to medical care: Experiences at LDS Hospital. *Medical Decision Making, 11*(Suppl. 4), S60–S65.

16. Kleefield, S., Churchill, W. W., & Laffel, G. (1991). Quality improvement in a hospital pharmacy department. *Quality Review Bulletin, 17*(5), 138–143.

17. Laffel, G. L., Berwick, D. M. (1993). Quality health care. *Journal of the American Medical Association, 270*(2), 254–255.

18. Quality connection. (1992). *News from the Institute for Healthcare Improvement, 1,* 8–9.

19. Heilig, S. (1990). The team approach to change: Organization-wide teamwork underlies quality enhancement process at University of Michigan Medical Center. *Healthcare Forum Journal,* (July/August), 19–22.

20. Koska, M. T. (1992). Using CQI methods to lower postsurgical wound infection rate. *Hospitals, 66*(9), 62–64.

21. Classen, D. C., Evans, R. S., Pestotnik, S. I., Horn, S. D., Menlove, R. L., & Burke, J. P. (1992). The timing of prophylactic administration of antibiotics and the risk of surgical-wound infection. *New England Journal of Medicine, 326,* 281–286.

22. Eisenberg, J. M. (1986). *Doctors' decisions and the costs of medical care.* Ann Arbor, MI: Health Administration Press.

23. McLaughlin, C. P., & Kaluzny, A. D. (1990). Total quality management in health: Making it work. *Health Care Management Review, 15*(3), 7–14.

24. Goldman, L. (1990). Changing physicians' behavior: The pot and the kettle. *New England Journal of Medicine, 322*(21), 1524–1525.

25. Soumerai, S. B., & Avorn, J. L. (1986). Economic and policy analysis of university-based drug "detailing." *Medical Care*, *24*, 313–331.

26. Lomas, J. (1991). Words without action? The production, dissemination, and impact of consensus recommendations. *Annual Review of Public Health*, *12*, 41–65.

27. Schroeder, S. A., Myers, L. P., McPhee, S. J., Showstack, J. A., Simborg, D. W., Chapman, S. A., & Leong, J. K. (1984). The failure of physician education as a cost containment strategy. *Journal of the American Medical Association*, *252*(2), 225–230.

28. Brennan, T. A., Lee, T. H., O'Neil, A., & Petersen, L. A. (n.d.). *Integrating providers into quality improvement: A pilot project at one hospital*. Unpublished manuscript. Brigham and Women's Hospital, Boston.

29. Feigenbaum, A. V. (1991). *Total quality control*. New York: McGraw-Hill.

30. Feigenbaum, A. V. (1951). *Total quality control*. New York: McGraw-Hill.

31. Nelson, E. C., & Berwick, D. M. (1989). The measurement of health status in clinical practice. *Medical Care*, *27*(Suppl. 3), S77–S90.

32. Mulley, A., Blumenthal, D., & Slavin, P. (1992). *Outcomes research: A potential force for constructive change in health care*. Unpublished manuscript.

33. Kravitz, R. L., Greenfield, S., Rogers, W., Manning, W. G., Jr., Zubkoff, M., Nelson, E. C., Tarlov, A. R., & Ware, J. E., Jr. (1992). Differences in the mix of patients among medical specialties and systems of care. Results from the medical outcomes study. *Journal of the American Medical Association*, *267*(12), 1617–1623.

34. Institute of Medicine. (1990). *Clinical practice guidelines*. Washington, DC: National Academy Press.

35. Gray, B. H. (1991). *The profit motive and patient care*. Cambridge, MA: Harvard University Press.

3

Continuous Quality Improvement and the Physician

Building Bridges with Outcomes Research

Sheldon Greenfield, M.D.

In the first part of this chapter I challenge the continuous quality improvement (CQI) movement by stating the following null hypothesis: if CQI leaders do not better appreciate the culture of physicians, they will not make any headway in their attempts to integrate CQI into the physician community. I also attempt to concretize, with case examples, the proposal to merge CQI with outcomes and quality research to enhance the integration and success of both. Those working in quality assessment and quality assurance have been attacked by the CQI movement because CQI asserts that the traditional forms of quality assessment and quality assurance have not worked, will not work, and have to be replaced. One reaction to this claim is simple acceptance and endorsement of the notion that quality assurance and quality assessment, as they originally were conceived and implemented, did not work. However, this acknowledgment may throw the baby out with the bathwater because evidence now suggests that without some of the traditional elements of quality assessment, particularly from the area of outcomes research, the CQI movement may not be able to sustain its progress in the physician community.

The questions raised in this chapter are concerned especially with whether CQI can be transferred to the health culture and have meaningful, rather than superficial, effects. When the Cadillac Division of the General Motors Corporation won the Baldridge Award for quality, the evidence used to evaluate Cadillac's merits was apparently far less exacting than the evidence normally required to prove the quality of clinical care in medicine. The Baldridge Award committee did not require that Cadillac be compared with its competitors in carefully controlled clinical trials that met the standards of peer-reviewed scholarly journals. And the quality measures applied to Cadillac would seem, at least to a physician, much less sophisticated than those applied to medical interventions. Car manufacturers must demonstrate that they can get their passengers from one place to another with greater comfort and safety than their competitors, such as in a Lexus or Mercedes. Medical care, in contrast, proves its worth through demonstrating symptom relief, improvement in quality of life, increased longevity, and enhanced patient satisfaction.

Getting Clear on the Goals of Improving Health Care Services

The different levels and types of evidence required to demonstrate quality in manufacturing as opposed to clinical settings are symptomatic of a translational problem that CQI faces in making its work relevant and useful in health care settings. Some advocates of CQI try to apply its methods in a simpleminded and direct way to health care. They often emphasize reduction in variation of health care processes as an end in itself. Physicians perceive this emphasis as either naive or worse—a threatening attempt to improve efficiency without attention to end results that matter most to patients and physicians. One way to avoid this misunderstanding, in my view, is through the marriage of outcomes research and CQI. Because of its focus on health care outcomes that really matter, outcomes research can provide CQI with a focus on goals that are meaningful to doctors. An emphasis on the attainment of comprehensive, health-related goals will facilitate the integration of continuous improvement into the physician culture.

To understand in more detail how a focus on outcomes will assist the CQI movement, it is useful to clarify some terms commonly used to characterize the health care delivery process: *efficiency, effectiveness,* and *quality.* All three are widely considered desirable attributes of health care. Each may be the objective of health care improvement efforts. Problems arise, however, when they are confused with one another. Part of the difficulty physicians have with CQI is that they perceive the methods of CQI as most appropriate to improving efficiency although CQI claims to be interested in quality.

Figures 3.1, 3.2, and 3.3 illustrate, using the example of patients entering a cardiac care unit, what I mean by these different attributes of the health care delivery process. *Efficiency,* as described in Figure 3.1, might be interpreted as how rapidly, consistently, and inexpensively actions are performed as a patient enters the coronary care unit. Much of CQI seems intent on reducing variation for the purpose of enhancing speed and consistency. It is hard to avoid the impression that reduction in expense, and thus enhanced efficiency, is really the chief concern underlying such efforts.

FIGURE 3.1 Efficiency

Care Processes

Admit to CCU and discharge within three days.
Administer thrombolysis.
Monitor for continuing chest pain.
Treat CHF if it develops.

Efficiency is how inexpensively, consistently, and rapidly these decisions and actions are carried out. Here is where variation can be minimized in the manufacturing sense.

In Figure 3.2, the term *effectiveness* is defined. As used here, effectiveness is attained when the proper treatment for a given patient with a given condition is chosen. For each step in the process of care, a maximally effective choice is available. In the administration of thrombolytics for patients with myocardial infarction, effectiveness is assessed through asking such questions as, Does thrombolysis reduce mortality from heart attacks? At what point in the natural history of the disease is thrombolysis most likely to have this effect? At what point is the effect greatest? How do the side effects compare with the benefits? In the light of this evidence, under what circumstances is thrombolysis an appropriate choice of therapy for heart attack victims? Most of the patient outcomes research teams (PORT) commissioned by the Agency for Health Care Policy and Research focus on such questions. They are concerned with relating choice of treatment with results or outcomes of care so that treatment choices can be improved. Often, they examine the costs of care as well, which allows them to assess not only effectiveness but also cost-effectiveness.

A third attribute of the health care delivery process, as illustrated in Figure 3.3, is its quality. The concept of quality is distinct from, though related to, both efficiency and effectiveness. It is a more comprehensive idea than either of these other attributes of health. *Quality* is achieved when the best attainable outcomes of care are realized. This accomplishment requires doing everything

FIGURE 3.2 Effectiveness

Care Processes

Admit to CCU and discharge within three days.
Administer thrombolysis.
Monitor for continuing chest pain.
Treat CHF if it develops.

Effectiveness is studying which discreet decisions work: should you use thrombolytics, which one, in which patients? It does not ask whether the processes of care were carried out well.

right: making the right choice, at the right time, with the proper execution, and with proper attention to all of the things that may affect the patient (patient education, comfort, compliance with care, the interaction of the various health problems the patient may have). Interestingly, we as physicians may identify the course of therapy that is highest in quality (in the sense of realizing the best outcomes for the patient) without completely understanding all of the reasons why this approach is so successful. In this sense, quality sometimes can be assessed with an incomplete grasp of efficiency or effectiveness. It also happens, not infrequently, that even when we do what seems effective and efficient, we do not maximize outcomes because we do not fully understand all aspects of the patient, his or her problems, and the applicable treatments.

A focus on any of these elements—efficiency, effectiveness, or quality—will improve the delivery of health care in one way or another, but it is useful to know exactly what the goals of the improvement effort are. Physicians generally will participate most willingly (regardless of the approach used) if they can identify and influence the goals of the improvement activities. If the desired result is to increase efficiency and save money by such means as decreasing length of stay, physicians may have limited interest because they may see it as an administrative issue and therefore in someone else's domain. If the goal in mind is to assess effectiveness,

FIGURE 3.3 Quality

Care Processes

Admit to CCU and discharge within three days.
Administer thrombolysis.
Monitor for continuing chest pain.
Treat CHF if it develops.

Quality is whether the aggregate of processes taken together lead to as good outcomes as is scientifically possible to obtain. This is where outcomes management comes in. Quality can be related to cost: if the outcomes are good and similar, can care be less expensive?

physicians generally will involve themselves to the extent that they will insist certain scientific standards of proof be demonstrated before they will accept any conclusions of the improvement activity. However, they may not care to participate directly because they understand that they cannot perform trials in their own practice settings. Alternatively, if improving quality is the purpose of the activity, physicians may demand involvement in the process of change because they see themselves as guardians of the global care of a patient. Physicians are in many ways well placed to make an assessment of whether quality has been attained because they are so closely in touch with the patients under care. Furthermore, they are responsible for the global outcomes of treatment. Indeed, a focus on quality in all of its aspects may be the most attractive approach for physicians because it relates most directly to their concerns and their perceived roles.

Outcomes research can help assess quality and thus potentiate CQI as an improvement methodology in a number of ways, described below. In the process, outcomes research can help make CQI more acceptable and relevant to physicians.

1. Establishment of Better Measures of Quality

Measures of outcomes, the end results of care, are complementary and often preferable to measures of process as indicators of quality. Sometimes, outcomes simply provide more information than process measures. For example, a low infection rate has been achieved by Intermountain Health Care's quality improvement efforts; the rate dropped from an already low level to an even lower level.[1] The "Six Hospital Study," however, has shown that mild infections have little measurable effect on outcomes of care six months after discharge.[2] Thus, reduction in infection rate may be a better measure of efficiency than of quality. In a similar vein, unpublished work demonstrates that certain aspects of the process of primary care—continuity, coordination, and comprehensiveness—were missing in certain settings[3] but that these deficiencies were not associated with any observed differences in two-year out-comes.[4] Total quality management (TQM) has a tendency to emphasize process improvement even when the evidentiary links to outcome have not been demonstrated. Emphasis on process improvement for its own sake may undermine the credibility of TQM if such limitations in its methods are not acknowledged and dealt with explicitly. Correspondingly, TQM will become more acceptable to physicians when its techniques for process improve-ment can be demonstrated to improve validated measures of out-come.

2. Improvement of Methods to Ensure Validity and Reliability

The outcomes movement also has the potential to improve the validity, reliability, and interpretability of methods currently advo-cated by practitioners of TQM. Control charts may be one exam-ple (see Chapter Two). Control charts are used often by industrial quality managers to monitor the performance of a process over time. Classically, industrial quality managers become concerned when a particular level of that attribute is exceeded—usually, when the level exceeds three standard deviations from the mean.

One problem with control charts as they have been applied to clinical situations, however, is that they seem to lack validity as indicators of the quality of care. As a result, they may be mislead-ing to naive physicians and outright offensive to more sophisticated clinicians. When an indicator used to monitor care in a population changes—such as blood sugar levels in diabetics or blood pressures in hypertensives—many factors may be at work. Characteristics of the patient group may have changed (case mix). So may have com-pliance with therapy by patients, the setting in which care is ren-dered, and the accuracy of the blood pressure or blood sugar measurement. To assess quality of care over time, the data that are plotted must be adjusted for these various factors. Unless it is cor-rected in this manner, the information displayed in the control chart may be misleading. It may be that industrial quality monitoring is a simpler business than quality monitoring in health care and that unadjusted data may have more value in those simpler settings. Alternatively, industrial quality managers may be sensitive to the potentially misleading nature of crude data and may take additional steps to confirm the validity of the changes observed on control charts. In other words, they may use the control chart as a form of exploratory data analysis that needs to be confirmed by more sophisticated techniques.

Whatever the case in industry, outcomes research has demonstrated time and again that many measures of process and outcome in clinical medicine are too sensitive and insufficiently specific to be relied on as the basis for action to improve quality.[5] Outcomes researchers rely on complex multivariate data analysis to improve quality indicators. Such techniques may offer useful guidance to CQI practitioners as they attempt to adapt industrial techniques to management of quality in health care settings. Perhaps such multivariate adjustment methods will have to be made more user-friendly before they can be applied in routine health care settings.

3. Setting Priorities for Improvement

The marriage of outcomes research with IQMS may enable quality managers to establish new quality improvement priorities that are more appealing to physicians and more important to the health of patients. As noted, outcomes research provides valid, reliable, and comprehensive measures of the health of patients. It thus allows and encourages physicians and policymakers to ask questions about which problems are most important in terms of their consequences for patients and which deserve highest priority in quality improvement activities. It is hard to avoid the impression that, in some of its applications, CQI loses the forest for the trees in quality management. CQI exercises seem at times to produce endless lists of processes that need improvement but offer no guidance on which should be addressed first. If CQI incorporated a formal method for relating process to outcome, then it might be possible to make more meaningful choices about which processes should be improved first. In this case, listing the many processes that are operating in a particular clinical sphere might be the first step in an orderly approach to quality improvement. Health outcomes such as quality of life and symptom relief might be targeted, whereas factors such as infection rates or patient satisfaction might not be as important. Generally, searching the literature for achievable outcomes and reaching consensus on how to measure such outcomes have not been, in my experience, major components of the CQI movement.

At a minimum, the CQI movement will be enhanced by including outcomes research. Outcomes researchers, in turn, will find enormous contributions from the CQI field because CQI can provide context, structure, and philosophy for the application of outcomes information.

When outcomes are included as part of CQI, some of the underlying conceptual issues related to the "treachery" or invalidity of outcomes must be addressed. This topic has been discussed in depth by Greenfield and Nelson[5]; issues raised include case mix adjustment, timing of assessment after treatment, prediction of the poor outcomes (events) enabling determination of appropriate patient group size, selection of optimal specific and sensitive outcomes, and developing "best guesses" pinpointing processes that affect the outcomes.

Synergy of Outcomes Research and CQI

A series of published studies demonstrates the effective and appropriate use of outcomes measures for continuous improvement. One example is Brent James's study that uses infection rate as the outcome. In addition, several mortality models have been developed for quality measurement, such as those of O'Connor[6] and Hannan[7] for cardiac care and coronary artery bypass procedures. These models effectively control for the confounding factors that affect outcomes and thereby allow inferences to be made about whether quality of care is a problem. Models of end-stage renal disease mortality are also available and reveal differences between sites that cannot easily be explained by case mix issues or by other confounding variables.

In a number of studies that successfully employed outcomes measures for quality improvement purposes, quality of life or functional status outcomes figured prominently. The results affect all patients who survive hospital care and are also critical outcomes for most outpatient care. Some of the studies presented below have moved beyond using outcomes methodology and consider the nature and amount of inputs. This extension enables a preliminary evaluation of the concept of value in health care because outcomes achieved can be associated with a given level of resources or input expended. Such a "next step" may assist continuous improvement within a health care institution by blending considerations of efficiency and quality. In general, efforts at continuous improvement in the 1990s will have to balance costs, quality, and satisfaction after controlling for case mix.

The first study I describe in detail is an unpublished pilot investigation[8] conducted at the Hospital Corporation of America (HCA). Notably, this work was conducted in an organization whose staff was actively attempting to implement the philosophy and methods of TQM. The chief individual leading the study was Eugene Nelson, who worked for HCA at that time. The project team was multidisciplinary and included insiders from the corporation, as well as outsiders. This delicately balanced team ensured that the study would balance the internal needs of HCA with the academic and policy perspectives of the researchers. The study focused on acute myocardial infarction (AMI) and drew patients from three small Southern hospitals whose administrations responded to mailed questionnaires that asked about the outcomes of AMI care, including mortality, functional status, level of angina, level of dyspnea, and satisfaction, all of which were measured eight weeks after discharge (see Table 3.1). Each outcome was adjusted for several factors: the severity of AMI was controlled through application of a standard measure; comorbidity was controlled by using a well-tested measure developed by an experienced research team; and congestive heart failure was controlled by examining chest X-rays and adjusting for gender and age. Total charges, ancillary charges, and length of stay were adjusted for the same variables. Information concerning case mix and process of care was obtained from medical records. In addition, administrative aspects of care, such as the time it took to get from the emergency room to the coronary care unit, were measured. Patients transferred from other facilities were excluded.

Table 3.1 illustrates the magnitude of differences in outcomes between hospitals that was evident after adjustment for all relevant factors. Hospital C had lower levels of angina and dyspnea among discharged patients, but physical function and emotional function were higher than at other hospitals. Furthermore, as shown in Table 3.2, Hospital C also had higher levels of resource use as reflected by length of stay, ancillary charges, and total charges. Overall, it appears that Hospital C invested more and got better results than its sister institutions. At the other two hospitals, outcomes were similar to each other, but length of stay was shorter in Hospital A than B. If Hospital C spent more money on amenities, this was not reflected in its patient satisfaction scores, which were high but equivalent to those of the other hospitals. Other complaints and problems were articulated in the patient satisfaction questionnaires, but overall the scores were equivalent.

What does this study show? It demonstrates that it is feasible to collect this kind of outcome information and to perform such a study with state-of-the-art measurement tools according to current concepts and theories. It also shows that it is possible to detect differences among hospitals in the "value" they offer through their care processes; providers and managers can use such information for continuous improvement, according to judgment or goals to balance cost and quality. However, these results are just the start of the process. In forthcoming steps, the data need to be reviewed, physician involvement must be increased, and the study results need to

TABLE 3.1 AMI Outcomes/Costs in Three Hospitals

	Hospital A			Hospital B			Hospital C		
	Unadjusted	Adjusted	(n)	Unadjusted	Adjusted	(n)	Unadjusted	Adjusted	(n)
Death	0.27	0.26	(48)	0.08	0.14	(40)	0.16	0.12	(45)
Angina	0.96	0.91	(28)	1.28	1.47	(25)	0.75	0.66	(24)
Dyspnea	1.04	1.20	(28)	1.76	1.90	(25)	0.67	0.89	(24)
Physical functioning	64.58	62.92	(28)	55.17	48.68	(25)	67.39	75.23	(23)
Emotional functioning	63.27	65.78	(27)	69.00	64.12	(25)	82.95	85.28	(22)
Overall satisfaction	80.95	81.86	(21)	81.67	80.54	(25)	82.99	83.16	(12)

Adjusted for age, gender, severity of MI, comorbidity, CHF by chest x-ray, history of coronary artery surgery.

TABLE 3.2 AMI Outcomes/Costs in Three Hospitals (Continued)

	Hospital A			Hospital B			Hospital C		
	Unadjusted	Adjusted	(n)	Unadjusted	Adjusted	(n)	Unadjusted	Adjusted	(n)
Total hospital charges	20,877	25,697	(48)	21,526	25,899	(40)	39,929	30,915	(45)
Total ancillary charges	8,116	11,256	(48)	8,292	11,198	(40)	22,156	16,219	(45)
Length of hospital stay	7.44	8.22	(48)	9.00	10.09	(40)	11.78	10.10	(45)
Return to work/normal practice	3.07	2.73	(22)	4.26	4.79	(59)	4.18	4.14	(17)
Major complication	0.43	0.43	(47)	0.30	0.39	(40)	0.51	0.42	(45)

Adjusted for age, gender, severity of MI, comorbidity, CHF by chest x-ray, history of coronary artery surgery.

be presented in a more user-friendly way to facilitate change where it appears necessary. Despite the study's limitations, however, it remains one of the first to combine the necessary elements on which improvements can be made by defining outcomes and charges and correspondingly adjusting for the defined patient population and case mix. Furthermore, although this study does not provide enough information about processes that might help explain variation in charges and outcomes, such information currently is being examined.

The next case study is the Medical Outcomes Study (MOS). A major thrust of MOS was to compare systems of care, specialties of care, levels of resource use, and kinds and levels of interpersonal care to each other and to determine the relationship between such factors and the outcomes produced (functional status, physiological measures, and death) over a two-year, and in some cases a four-year, period. An initial cross-sectional study was completed in 1986 with more than twenty thousand patients who constituted a 70-percent sample of patients who came into the offices of more than five hundred practitioners. For 96 percent of the patients, the doctors provided clinical information by using a short form. An approximate 10-percent sample then was followed for at least two years, with a physical examination and laboratory work performed at both the beginning and end of that period. This study was the largest study of office practice of its kind ever conducted. Its relevance here is the information it provided that relates inputs of care to outcomes. The study examined whether some systems of care or certain specialties use more resources or different types of resources and, if so, what relationship such differences in practice had to outcomes for their patients. Conversely, it examined whether certain systems or specialties were more efficient because they produced the same outcomes at lower rates of resource use.

Data on utilization have been presented elsewhere and are displayed in Table 3.3.[9] These data show that patients cared for in indemnity, fee-for-service, solo, or single-specialty practices tend to have higher utilization rates of hospitals and drugs than patients of multispecialty groups. HMO patients have the lowest rates of resource use. Not yet reported are the outcome data. Preliminary analyses for more than six hundred hypertension patients, about 40 percent of the total longitudinal sample, indicate no differences between systems of care with respect to physiological or functional outcomes over this two-year period.[4] The measured physiological outcomes included systolic blood pressure and diastolic blood pressure calculated both as means for the whole group and as reductions for those patients who initially had high blood pressures. In addition, the study tracked measures of the signs and symptoms of congestive heart failure, any changes in these measures over two years, and measures of functional status and quality of life as assessed by the Short Form 36. If these data can be assessed as planned, it will be possible to study value of care in alternative settings as measured by input required to achieve a given level of outcome. Such evaluations can proceed for these systems and for any units that have at least several hundred patients. It should be possible to assess the outcomes of treatment for common diseases managed in office practices, after adjusting for factors that independently could affect both physiology and function.

For continuous improvement purposes, these types of information do not specifically identify which processes are associated with excess expenditures or which processes do not seem related to improved outcomes. In fact, process measures were relatively crude, and as in the myocardial infarction study previously described, it will be necessary to link key processes to key outcomes in order to address those areas of each that can be influenced and improved. This study also found some satisfaction differences between systems of care.[10] With such data, managers can begin improving those systems of care that have higher use rates or poorer satisfaction ratings, controlling for outcomes of care. Resulting changes may reduce costs, improve quality, or both.

The diabetes PORT study[11] provides a third example in which researchers are trying to link resource use and outcomes of care. This project concentrates on one disease that is commonly managed in

TABLE 3.3 Comparison of Patient Mix and Unadjusted and Adjusted Utilization Rates for Six Indicators Among the Five Systems.*

	HMO	MSG-PP	Solo/SSG-PP	MSG-FFS	Solo/SSG-FFS	P
Patient Mix Indicators						
Mean age, y	45.0	38.6	42.4	48.8	49.2	<.0001
Educational level, y	13.6	13.6	13.9	13.1	13.6	.001
Number of chronic diseases per patient	0.93	0.69	0.81	0.93	1.10	<.0001
General health perception (0-100 scale)	68.2	71.1	69.0	67.1	67.6	.02
Unadjusted Use Rates						
% Hospitalized	4.43	3.60 (81)	4.35 (98)	5.98 (135)	8.01 (181)†	<.01
Office visits per patient per y	4.35	4.35 (100)	4.21 (97)	4.29 (99)	4.70 (108)	<.001
Prescription drugs per patient	1.31	1.18 (90)	1.21 (92)	1.49 (114)	1.69 (129)†	<.05
% Patients having tests per visit‡	43.9	37.4 (85)§	47.7 (109)	41.3 (94)	47.4 (108)	<.05
Mean value of tests per visit‡	26.30	20.50 (78)§	25.70 (98)	23.30 (89)	28.50 (108)†	<.05
Mean value of tests per y‡	105.70	82.40 (78)	94.90 (90)	91.10 (86)	122.20 (116)	<.01
Adjusted Use Rates						
% Hospitalized	4.93	4.24 (86)	4.92 (100)	5.58 (113)	6.94 (141)§	<.05
Office visits per patient per y	4.68	4.73 (101)	4.33 (93)	4.17 (89)†	4.30 (92)§	<.001
Prescription drugs per patient	1.37	1.45 (106)	1.32 (96)	1.46 (107)§	1.53 (112)†	<.01
% Patients having tests per visit‡	43.8	38.4 (88)	48.0 (110)	42.1 (96)	47.0 (107)	.06
Mean value of tests per visit‡	26.10	22.40 (86)	26.50 (102)	24.50 (94)	27.40 (105)	<.01
Mean value of tests per patient per y‡	116.40	103.70 (89)	110.00 (95)	91.70 (79)†	113.80 (98)	<.05

*HMO indicates health maintenance organization; MSG-PP, multispecialty group-prepaid; Solo/SSG-PP, solo practice/single-speciality group-prepaid; MSG-FFS, multispecialty group–fee-for-service; and Solo/SSG-FFS, solo practice/single-specialty group–fee-for-service Numbers in parentheses are the ratios of that system's use rate to that of the HMO, which equals 100. Sample size varies by type of use: for hospitalizations, 9435; for office visits, 18353; for prescription drugs, 18573; for tests and procedures, 18269. Of the total number of patients studied, 37% were in HMOs, 10% MSG-PP, 12% Solo/SSG-PP, 6% MSG-FFS, and 34% Solo/SSG-FFS.

†P≤.01; ‡Mean value of tests or procedures; §P≤.05.

Source: Greenfield, S. (1992). Variations in resource utilization among medical specialities and systems of care. *Journal of the American Medical Association, 267*(12), 1624-1630. Copyright © 1992, American Medical Association. Reprinted by permission.

primary care settings and that is protean in its health effects: diabetes affects all organ systems except the lungs. For the diabetes PORT, utilization and expenditure data are available at the health plan level (from Group Health Cooperative of Puget Sound [GHC] and Tufts Associated Health Plan [TAHP] in particular). In addition, an administrative database is available and can be linked to clinical data such as laboratory values and patient reports. This linkage provides a more comprehensive source of data from which processes, outcomes, expenditures, and utilization information can be matched to track achievement of different improvement goals and associated costs: reduction in the number of amputations in hospitalizations for foot care, reduction of renal disease, reduction of heart disease, and reduction of eye disease.

In the diabetes PORT, the unit of analysis is at the physician level. Each physician follows at least twenty patients, which enables some analysis by physician after adjusting for case mix. By obtaining information about each individual patient, case mix adjustments can be more accurate because records will include information about certain values obtained from the administrative database and medical records will be used only minimally, if at all. Ideally, this approach will enable adjustment for case mix and analyses by individual physicians or by small group practices to assess outputs of care. These outcomes may include functional status and physiological indicators (for example, hemoglobin A1C). This study also will enable use of combinations of generic and disease-specific measures along with physiological measures and mortality rates to produce an array of indicators that may be sensitive and specific to treatments and that may effectively link processes of care to relevant outcomes.

The final case example was undertaken in a continuous improvement environment by a team of researchers (Lawrence Gottlieb, Greenfield, and others) at the Harvard Community Health Plan (HCHP). The aim of the study was to test the effect of using guidelines on patient outcomes. In other words, this study was designed to evaluate whether guidelines improved or worsened patient outcomes or kept outcomes constant while reducing resource use. For patients with dyspepsia, the study assessed whether the processes of care, as recorded in patient charts, were influenced by guidelines and whether changes in processes of care were associated with different outcomes.

Illustrated in Table 3.4 are the utilization results that correspond to the practice guidelines for dyspepsia. Here, utilization does not exactly mirror the guidelines. For example, in the guidelines group, upper GI series was not recommended. Instead, the failure of empirical treatment, or "watchful waiting," results in a referral to gastroenterology. However, the content of these guidelines is relatively unimportant; the major reason for showing these data is to illustrate how resource utilization can be related to outcomes as shown in Table 3.5.

If one were to review these materials from a continuous improvement point of view, one might easily be pleased with the way expenditures relate to outcomes. Alternatively, one might ask whether expenditures could be decreased by reducing referral for ultrasounds and upper GI series, and interest might be piqued in further analysis of the actual guidelines to see how rigorously they were followed and whether compliance has any relationship to outcomes among a larger number of patients. In response to such additional analyses, guidelines could be changed to alter expenditure patterns and to assess whether outcomes could be improved.

These four case studies provide different examples of the ways outcomes can be integrated into a continuous improvement environment by studying (1) processes as they affect outcomes and (2) resource use in relation to benefit. Admittedly, these studies are crude, and they do have important limitations. Primarily, they were not repeated; thus, they do not provide evidence for patterns of continuous improvement. A second limitation is that none of these studies provided sufficient detail about processes to point directly at opportunities to modify these processes for the purpose of quality improvement. Third, participation of physicians in these studies was uneven. Fourth, each study had methodological or

TABLE 3.4 Use Patterns of Patients of Control and Experimental Physician Groups for All Patients with Dyspepsia[†]

Process	Control (n = 43)	Experimental (n = 54)	Mean difference (± 95% CI)
Referral to gastroenterology	11.6	18.5	-6.9 (–21.0, 7.2)
Upper GI series	25.6	24.1	1.5 (-15.8, 18.8)
Endoscopy	4.7	3.7	1.0 (-7.1, 26.3)
Gallbladder ultrasound	27.9	18.5	9.4 (-7.5, 26.3)
CT scan and/or abdominal x-ray	11.6	9.3	2.3 (-10.0, 14.6)
Amylase	34.9	42.6	-7.7 (-2.7.1, 11.7)
Liver function tests	46.5	51.9	-5.4 (-25.4, 14.6)

[†]Percentage of patients having each service.

measurement flaws that could be improved. Combined with results from other studies, however, these studies demonstrate that relatively sophisticated data on outcomes are interpretable, feasible to collect, and meaningful to use. In addition, the studies show that outcomes data can assist in identifying processes that need further study to accomplish improvements highly valued by physicians, institution administrators, and patients.

Outcomes research and its methods, therefore, can contribute to the effectiveness of CQI in the medical environment through a number of routes. It can help demonstrate the relationships between processes of care and outcomes. It can focus attention on specific processes that matter most to physicians and patients. In this way, it can assist physicians and administrators to meet the needs of patients. It can make TQM meaningful to doctors. The merging of outcomes research with continuous improvement has the potential, therefore, to facilitate the implementation of TQM in health care organizations.

TABLE 3.5 Patient Health Outcome Measures by Physician Group[*†]

Outcome	Number of Items	Control mean ($n = 43$)	Experimental mean ($n = 54$)	Mean difference (± 95% CI)
Physical function	10	86.2 (3.7)	83.4 (3.4)	2.8 (–7.1, 12.7)
Role function	4	74.2 (6.3)	80.4 (5.5)	-6.2 (-22.6, 10.2)
Pain	2	66.0 (4.2)	72.0 (3.5)	-6.0 (-16.6, 4.6)
Mental health index	5	69.9 (3.3)	67.9 (2.7)	2.0 (-6.3, 10.3)
Energy/vitality	4	57.1 (3.1)	55.0 (2.6)	2.1 (-5.8, 10.0)
Role function emotional	3	79.2 (5.6)	74.2 (5.2)	5.0 (-10.0, 20.0)
General health perceptions	5	68.8 (2.8)	68.4 (2.3)	0.4 (-6.6, 7.4)
Social function	2	82.3 (3.3)	84.3 (2.8)	-2.0 (-10.4, 6.4)
Health transition	1	51.4 (3.9)	50.9 (3.3)	0.5 (-9.5, 10.5)
Satisfaction	10	66.0 (3.0)	65.6 (2.5)	0.5 (-7.2, 8.0)
Prevention of food consumption due to pain	1	65.4 (5.0)	68.3 (4.1)	-2.9 (-15.5, 9.7)
Decrease in normal daily activity due to pain	1	72.0 (3.8)	78.4 (3.3)	-6.4 (-16.2, 3.4)
Decrease in social activity due to pain	1	73.8 (4.3)	80.2 (3.7)	-6.4 (-17.5, 4.7)

* Adjusted for within physician correlations.
† Table entries are means with standing errors in parentheses.

Notes

1. Classen, D. C., Evans, R. S., Pestotnik, S. I., Horn, S. D., Menlove, R. L., & Burke, J. P. (1992). The timing of prophylactic administration of antibiotics and the risk of surgical-wound infection. *New England Journal of Medicine, 326,* 281–286.

2. Cleary, P. D., Greenfield, S., Mulley, A. G., Pauker, S. G., Schroeder, S. A., Wexler, L., & McNeil, B. J. (1991). Variations in length of stay and outcomes for six medical and surgical conditions in Massachusetts and California. *Journal of the American Medical Association, 266,* 73–79.

3. Safran, D. G., Tarlov, A. R., & Rogers, W. H. (1994). Primary care performance in fee-for-service and prepaid health care systems. *Journal of the American Medical Association, 271*(20), 1579–1586.

4. Greenfield, S., Rogers, W. H., Mangotich, M., Carney, M. F., & Tarlov, A. R. (in press). Do systems and specialties with higher utilization rates achieve better outcomes for patients with hypertension? Results from the Medical Outcomes Study. *Journal of the American Medical Association.*

5. Greenfield, S., & Nelson, E. (1992). Recent developments and future issues in the use of health status assessment measures in clinical settings. *Medical Care, 30*(5S), 23–41.

6. O'Connor, G. T., Plume, S. K., Olmstead, E. M., Coffin, L. H., et al. (1991). A regional prospective study of in-hospital mortality associated with coronary artery bypass grafting. *Journal of the American Medical Association, 266*(6), 803–809.

7. Hannan, E. L., Kilburn, H., Jr., O'Donnell, J. F., et al. (1990). Adult open heart surgery in New York State: An analysis of risk factors and hospital mortality rates. *Journal of the American Medical Association, 264,* 2768–2774.

8. Nelson, E., Cleary, P. D., Larson, C., & Greenfield, S. (1994). *The determination of costs in relation to eight-week outcomes in AMI patients: A comparison of three community hospitals.* Manuscript submitted for publication.

9. Greenfield, S., Nelson, E., Manning, W. G., Zubkoff, M., Rogers, W., et al. (1992). Variations in resource utilization among medical specialties and systems of care: Results from the Medical Outcomes Study. *Journal of the American Medical Association, 267*(12), 1624–1630.

10. Rubin, H. R., Bandek, B., Rogers, W. H., Kosinski, M., McHorney, C., & Ware, J. E., Jr. (1993). Patients' ratings of outpatient visits in different practice settings. *Journal of the American Medical Association, 270*(7), 835–840.

11. Greenfield, S., Kaplan, S. H., Silliman, R. A., Sullivan, L., Manning, W., et al. (1994). The uses of outcomes research for medical effectiveness, quality of care, and reimbursement in Type II diabetes. *Diabetes Care, 17*(1), 32–39.

4

Industrial Quality Management Science and Outcomes Research

Responses to Unwanted Variation in Health Outcomes and Decisions

Albert G. Mulley, Jr., M.D.

This is a time of sweeping change for quality assurance and improvement in health care. The stimuli for change are multiple. One is the desire to preserve quality of care in the face of a radical restructuring of the health care economy aimed at reducing costs of services. A second is the apparent opportunity provided by new approaches to quality improvement pioneered in industry as part of its response to international competition. These new approaches sometimes are labeled "industrial quality management science" (IQMS) or "total quality management" (TQM).

A third and perhaps most potent cause for change in quality management in the United States is the accumulating evidence of two kinds of unexplained variations that may constitute threats to quality: (1) differences in outcomes of care when seemingly similar patients receive seemingly similar treatments from different providers and (2) differences in the types of treatments prescribed by providers for seemingly similar patients with the same problems. The documentation of such variations in outcomes and treatment has formed a primary stimulus for outcomes research, a field that is central to current efforts to improve quality of care and service.

The purpose of this chapter is to provide some perspective on the source and nature of this unexplained variation in health care today and to describe a model for responding constructively to that variation. A major advantage of this proposed model is its ability to preserve differences in care that may be desirable (because they reflect the unique needs and expectations of individual patients) while reducing the variation that may be undesirable (and that constitutes a threat to quality of care). Another purpose of this chapter is to demonstrate that both outcomes research and IQMS have valuable contributions to make in responding to unexplained variation in the outcomes and treatments provided to patients. In fact, their contributions are complementary and mutually reinforcing.

Evidence of Variation in Outcomes and Practices in Health Care

Differences in the results of care—such as mortality and complication rates—after application of similar procedures, treatments, or hospitalizations have been examined and reported by health services researchers for decades.[1] Much effort has been expended in trying to explain such variation in outcomes. For some conditions and procedures, the volume of care provided by a given hospital or physician has proven to be a strong predictor of outcome.[1-3] Such findings attracted little attention from providers, policymakers, or patients, however, until the highly publicized release of hospital mortality data by the Health Care Financing Administration in 1986.[4] This release was followed quickly by release of statewide surgical mortality rates for institutions in Pennsylvania, New York, and elsewhere. The validity of inferences drawn from the comparative outcome rates was questioned, and these questions were often well justified. But in a newly consumer-oriented health care marketplace, the data could not be dismissed. Patients and payers, sensitized to possible differences in quality, sought "centers of excellence." Providers, many for the first time, examined the outcomes of their care in an effort to support claims of excellence or, at least, to deflect any perceptions about poor quality of care.

At the same time, the medical profession has been trying to understand the variation in health care treatments or practices among different geographical areas.[7-11] The practice variation phenomenon has been interpreted differently by different stakeholders in the health care system: as evidence for underuse due to poor access or provider bias[10-12]; as evidence of poor quality of care reflected in overuse or underuse[13]; and as evidence for provider-induced demand for services contributing to uncontrolled increases in health care costs.

Sources of Variation in Outcomes and Practices

In thinking about variation in outcomes of care and health care practices, it is helpful to pause a moment to reflect on exactly what is varying and what the sources of or reasons for that variation might be. This reflection will provide some assistance in understanding how both outcomes research and IQMS may be helpful in preserving variation that is desirable and in eliminating variation that is undesirable, thus improving quality of care.

At the risk of oversimplification, one can describe the provision of care to an individual patient with a particular problem as consisting of two closely related processes: (1) a process of deciding what care to provide and (2) a process of providing that care. In the first process, quality consists of a good decision: choosing the right procedure or treatment. In the second process, quality consists of proper performance or execution: providing the right care right. On the one hand, when we as doctors observe variation in the types of treatments provided to apparently similar patients, variation in the process of decision is responsible. On the other hand, when we observe differences in outcomes of care for similar patients provided the same types of treatments for the same conditions, presumably variation in the execution of care is responsible.

The sources of variation in processes of decision and performance are multiple. Some of these sources are threats to quality, others actually may improve it, and the aim of quality improvement should be to counteract the former, not the latter. For example, in the process of decision, patients' personal preferences for alternative outcomes achievable with different treatments may vary from one individual to another. These differences in preferences should result in variation in decision making that is appropriate and that improves quality by ensuring that outcomes will meet patients' needs and expectations. Physicians also may have strong personal preferences for one form of treatment or another, and as illustrated below, such preferences clearly explain some of the observed variation in practice from one geographical location to another. When such preferences are based on physicians' personal bias, habit, or unexamined assumptions, rather than on scientific data and reasoning, they may constitute an unwanted source of variation and a threat to quality of care.

Differences in the outcomes of care after application of the same procedure may result also from wanted and unwanted sources of variation. Unwanted sources of variation include differences in the technical skill of the physicians, nurses, or technicians or the level of organization and teamwork displayed by these personnel. Desired variation may be introduced as part of systematic experimentation to improve the performance of care (for example, in an effort to develop new and better surgical techniques).

Roles of Outcomes Research and IQMS in Improving Decision and Performance Quality

Because both IQMS and outcomes research are relatively new fields, they are not yet fully understood by many health care policymakers or even by many experts on quality of care. The tendency among some observers has been to see these two bodies of knowledge as separate and different approaches to improving health care quality. However, a brief examination of these two approaches to quality shows that they share similar aims, similar values, and many similar techniques. Furthermore, they tend to emphasize somewhat different approaches to quality improvement, and thus they may be stronger in combination than either would be alone.

Outcomes Research

Outcomes research is a diverse and evolving body of knowledge whose purpose is to improve quality of care and to reduce its costs by learning from observed variation in outcomes of care. As previously noted, the aims and methods of outcomes research reflect to some degree its origins in the variation phenomenon, which has done so much to alert physicians, purchasers, and policymakers to deficiencies in quality of care and service.

Outcomes research asks and answers questions of the following type:

1. How should the results of care be measured? In particular, how should we as physicians measure the more elusive dimensions of outcomes of care: effects on patients' functional status, effects on quality of life, and effects on patient satisfaction?

2. By using the best available measures, what can we learn about and from the results of care provided in different settings, by different providers, or to different patients? In particular, can we learn anything from the variation in results of care that may point to opportunities to make better choices regarding treatment?

3. Where the results of care do not vary across different circumstances, in which setting is the provision of care most efficient?

One important dimension of outcomes research is its emphasis on learning about and responding to patients' wishes and preferences for their treatment. This orientation reflects a number of developments: improved techniques for measuring subjective outcomes of care that patients may care a great deal about; patients' increasing desire to be included more in the medical decision-making process; a recognition that including patients in decision making may have an independent effect on outcomes; and an appreciation that patients may provide data that can assist in measuring the quality of care.

Outcomes research can contribute to improving the quality of care in a great variety of ways. Perhaps most important, it provides valid, reliable, and credible technologies for measuring something that physicians and patients care about in regard to the output of health care processes: the effect of those processes on health status in all of its dimensions. The effect of health care on health status is a fundamental attribute of quality, and outcomes research provides scientifically sound approaches to measuring that quality attribute.

Once available and applied, such quality indicators can be of enormous practical use. By revealing variation in quality, they can motivate providers whose patients experience poorer results to ask why their results are not as good as those of colleagues and to change behavior in response. Outcome measures also make it possible to set priorities for improvement so that scarce resources can be used to maximum effect. Where variation in outcomes is substantial, the opportunity for improvement by reducing that variation may be greater, all else being equal. Similarly, outcomes research highlights the question of which outcomes patients and doctors value most and whether improvement activities should focus on processes associated with the most highly valued outcomes. A further contribution of outcomes research to quality management has been to encourage the inclusion of patients and their preferences in the process of medical decision making.

Industrial Quality Management Science

Industrial quality management science (IQMS) is an eclectic blend of concepts and techniques drawn from diverse disciplines, including statistics, operations research, industrial engineering, sociology, management theory, and practical experience with quality management. Like the field of outcomes research, it is difficult to describe briefly, but the following tenets are among its most important:

1. Quality must be measured and measured accurately to be improved.

2. Continuous improvement in quality results from a never-ending effort to improve the processes of production and service in a health care organization.

3. Process improvement often results from understanding, controlling, or eliminating sources of variation in processes of production.

4. Quality improvement requires the involvement of personnel at every level of an organization: quality is everyone's business.

5. The customer is the ultimate judge of quality. Quality improvement requires a total commitment to meeting the needs and expectations of the customer.

6. Organizational leadership is essential to quality improvement.

The first three of these tenets capture some of the scientific content of TQM. To improve quality, it should be measured, its determinants characterized, and those determinants manipulated to achieve improvement. Variation in the process of production is often a source of quality problems and should be reduced.

The last three of these tenets capture some of the "softer" or more philosophical elements in TQM and reflect the experience of Deming, Juran, and others who have tried over the years to get industrial organizations to embrace scientific methods of quality improvement. After decades of trying to get real-world organizations to embrace scientific methods of quality improvement, advocates of such methods realized that science was not enough to make human beings and their organizations' policymakers behave differently. Certain kinds of managerial and attitudinal changes were necessary as well.

Like outcomes research, IQMS can contribute to quality in a number of ways. It shares with outcomes research a commitment to measuring quality as a starting point for quality improvement. In fact, if outcomes are important to quality in health care, then IQMS researchers would agree wholeheartedly with outcomes researchers that accurate measurement of outcomes is critical to quality improvement.

IQMS also shares with outcomes research a deep interest in finding out what customers (in this case, patients) want and in using that information to improve the performance of the system. Practitioners of IQMS anticipated seventy years ago the current emphasis of outcomes researchers on involving patients in decisions about health care.

Furthermore, IQMS is concerned, like outcomes research, with learning from and controlling sources of variation in the process of production that may cause undesirable variation in outcomes (reducing quality). In fact, variation in quality and processes of production was an important stimulus to the development of IQMS, as it was to the development of outcomes research.

Despite these remarkable areas of overlap with outcomes research, IQMS does have one important difference that gives it complementary strengths. As a practical matter, IQMS has concerned itself much more than outcomes research with developing methods for characterizing and continuously improving the performance of the processes of production in large organizations. This focus on process improvement reflects a firm conviction, based in practical experience, that process improvement results in quality improvement. As a result, IQMS has perfected methods for understanding in minute detail how processes work, where they fail, and how the scientific method can be harnessed to make them function better.

Thus, IQMS can be viewed as specializing in finding ways to improve the performance or execution of processes care. In contrast, outcomes research has tended to make its major contributions by correlating outcomes with treatment choices. These apparently

TABLE 4.1 Attributes of IQMS and Outcomes Research

Observation:	Outcome variation	Practice variation
Examples:	Hospital mortality Surgical mortality	Hospitalization rates Surgery rates
Causes:	Variation in processes	Variation in clinical decisions
Responses:	IQMS	Outcomes research
Goal:	Improve performance quality	Improve decision quality

different areas of concentration in the two fields have led to the further impression that outcomes research is best suited to improving decision quality in health care, whereas IQMS is best suited to improving performance quality.

The rationales for IQMS and outcomes research as discussed below are presented in Table 4.1.

To illustrate these similarities and differences between outcomes research and IQMS and between decision quality and performance quality and to set the stage for developing a model for continuous improvement in health care, it is useful to consider the opportunities for quality improvement associated with two common clinical conditions: coronary artery disease and breast cancer. As a subtheme, the ensuing discussion also makes clearer one of the most important similarities between IQMS and outcomes research: their commitment to including the patient and the patients' preferences in defining and improving quality of care.

Performance Quality and Decision Quality: Ischemic Heart Disease and Breast Cancer

The Patient's Perspective

Consider two lives. A sixty-six-year-old male retired college professor has had chest tightness with physical exertion or emotional stress for the past two years. It is moderately well controlled by medical treatments, but he has episodes predictably when he plays tennis or jogs. He sometimes has chest pain when he and his wife engage in sexual activity. The predictable discomfort, or angina, can be avoided if he takes nitroglycerin before the precipitating activity, but this works only about half the time. The angina gradually has become more limiting with regard to both physical and psychological functioning. A coronary angiogram was performed just two weeks ago to determine whether the coronary disease might be amenable to and warrant either surgery or another procedure. The angiogram showed that two coronary arteries were partially blocked. Although the blockages were not in life-threatening locations, they were severe enough to explain his symptoms. What should he do?

Similarly, consider the situation faced by a forty-two-year-old woman who has just learned she has breast cancer. She is a lawyer, a wife, and a mother of two small children. The tumor was discovered after she felt a small lump in her right breast. Mammography showed a suspicious lesion with a diameter just over one centimeter; needle biopsy confirmed that she had cancer. No evidence of tumor spread to lymph nodes or elsewhere was found. Should she have her breast removed, or should she have the breast irradiated after removal of the tumor? If surgery confirms the small tumor size and absence of tumor spread, should she take hormonal therapy or chemotherapy to reduce risk of cancer recurrence?

Clearly, life has been changed for each of these patients by the diagnosis of coronary disease or breast cancer, and it will be changed further by treatment. Both the man with coronary disease and the woman with breast cancer face difficult, complex decisions at a time when they may be least able to think rationally or to bear decision-making responsibility. We as physicians know that the breast cancer diagnosis evokes anger, a sense of isolation, irrational guilt, and most of all, vulnerability. Many of the same reactions are evident in men and women with coronary disease. The visualization of coronary blockages is tangible proof of the risk of heart attack, which always includes risk of death. This mix of emotions may make it very difficult to be involved in decision making. Under these circumstances, some patients have a strong desire to rely on the doctor, to trust that professional knowledge and technical skill can ensure that the right thing will be done right.

Outcome Variation, Practice Variation, and Implications for Quality

Will the right thing be done? Practice and outcome variation related to treatment of both conditions—angina and breast cancer—suggest otherwise. For the patient with stable or gradually worsening symptoms of ischemic heart disease, there are three alternative approaches: (1) continued medical therapy, (2) coronary artery bypass graft surgery (CABG), and (3) percutaneous coronary angioplasty (PTCA). Rates of CABG have been increasing for the past two decades as the procedure has been offered to older and more severely ill patients. Since its widespread clinical introduction in 1983, PTCA use has increased dramatically, substituting for medical therapy more often than for CABG.[14] Wide variations in the rates of death and other outcomes following CABG and PTCA have been documented, as has an association between volume of procedures performed by the surgeon or cardiologist and the volume of procedures performed at the hospital. In New York State, for example, adjusted mortality rates for patients after CABG were more than fivefold higher when the procedure was performed by a low-volume surgeon in a low-volume hospital than when performed by a high-volume surgeon in a high-volume hospital.[3] Since the initial publication of CABG mortality rates, statewide rates in New York have improved because of either improvement in the quality of care or changes in patient selection.[15] Similar variability in CABG outcome rates among hospitals in northern New England prompted the systematic application of some of the tools of IQMS in a collaboration that included all hospitals in the region at which CABG is performed. The processes used to deliver care to CABG patients were scrutinized carefully; associations between variations in execution of those processes and quality were sought.

But even if application of IQMS can help improve quality of care by controlling variation in the performance of CABG, PTCA, or medical therapy, how do doctors know when and whether each alternative is the right thing to do? Evidence is ample for discretion and differing opinions; these interventions have been shown to vary widely in use from one geographical area to another. In 1981, CABG rates among Medicare beneficiaries in thirteen geographical regions ranged from 70 to 230 per 1,000.[8] In 1982, the adjusted rate for inhabitants of greater New Haven was twice that for inhabitants of greater Boston.[16] PTCA rates show similar variation and, in some studies, have been shown to be positively associated with CABG rates. For the man with coronary disease, these findings suggest that how he is treated could depend more on where he lives or who cares for him than on who he is and what he cares about. This variation in practice strongly suggests the need to focus on the quality of decision making about treatment alternatives—on decision quality.

The cost associated with increasing use of PTCA and CABG, together with the variation in rates in different geographical areas, has led to the development of guidelines by professional organizations, including the American College of Cardiology.[20,24] But these guidelines are complex and require simultaneous consideration of multiple clinical variables, a difficult task for even the most knowledgeable clinician. Measures of appropriateness for both CABG and PTCA have been developed and used by payers to authorize or deny payment for procedures.[18,19] These criteria reflect judgments of expert clinicians, working with a modified delphi process and a common literature review, ranking hundreds of combinations of clinical variables on a nine-point numerical scale. Agreement among panel members and between panels using the same information and processes has been low. Using a generous definition of *agreement*, panelists considering appropriateness of CABG agreed in characterizing 30 percent of indications on the first round. Agreement after conferring and revising ratings increased to 40 percent. When U.S. and U.K. panels independently developed appropriateness criteria that subsequently were applied retrospectively to the same cases, 14 percent and 34 percent, respectively, were deemed inappropriate by the two criteria sets.[20] When such criteria are applied to cases in different geographical areas that have high and low use rates, no differences in levels of appropriateness are found. This finding may be explained by the substantial overlap in appropriate indications for alternative treatments. Clearly, such an approach offers only tentative answers to questions about which intervention is right for the retired professor or for any other particular patient with coronary disease. In fact, the danger is that such criteria can obscure the existing professional uncertainty and foster inattention to the patient's role in the decision-making process.

A patient outcomes research team (PORT) funded by the Agency for Health Care Policy and Research has developed an agenda to use existing databases to refine estimates of outcome probabilities for different patient subgroups treated with each modality. Establishing such relationships between the use of a treatment and its results clearly could assist the decision-making process and improve decision quality. The PORT is also developing measures of how patients value the outcomes associated with coronary disease and its treatment to better inform decisions about which treatment is right for specific patients. Knowledge of such preferences can help preserve desired variation in the process of decision making. As such, the work of the PORT provides an example of outcomes research aimed at determining the right decision for each individual patient experiencing a medical problem.[28]

Similar problems and concerns arise from the epidemiology of health care for women with early-stage breast cancer. American women face a one-in-nine chance of developing breast cancer in their lifetimes.[22] Fortunately, major advances in our understanding of breast cancer treatment have occurred in the last decade. Multiple clinical trials have demonstrated that either of two forms of primary therapy—breast-conserving surgery (BCS) followed by radiation, *or* mastectomy—afford women equivalent survival.[23-26] Furthermore, new analyses indicate that the beneficial effect of adjuvant therapy (hormone therapy or chemotherapy following primary therapy of the breast tumor) on survival and recurrence is applicable to more women and is more durable than previously believed.[27,28]

Despite this new knowledge about treatment, unexplained variations in patterns of treatment have been demonstrated repeatedly for patients of differing age, race, geographical region, and hospital type. These findings suggest the need to examine the process of decision making in breast cancer care and the possibility that decision quality could be improved. For example, 1988 rates of BCS varied more than threefold among regions of the United States—from 11.5 percent in the East South Central region to 40.2 percent in New England.[29] In the Medicare population, where even wider variations have been demonstrated among different state populations, patients treated at large, urban, or teaching hospitals and hospitals with radiation centers were more likely to undergo BCS.[30]

Variation in treatment decisions for use of adjuvant therapy are less well documented. But here, too, despite multiple NIH-sponsored consensus conferences, each of which produced cogent recommendations, there is reason to be concerned about the quality of decision making.[31-33] Different doctors make different recommendations, especially for low-risk women. Explanations for these patterns of care are not well understood. Patient preferences for alternative approaches to breast cancer treatment may be important, but the degree to which those preferences vary systematically by age, race, or geographical location is not well studied. The striking geographical variation in choices of surgical treatment, which is not likely explained by differences in patient preferences, suggests an important role for variable professional opinions as determinants of practice patterns. Several reports support this hypothesis.[34,35] Again, from the patient's perspective, the real concern is that treatment decisions may not reflect personal values and preferences unless the decision process includes the patient in a meaningful way.

Patients' Decision-Making Role

Practice variation suggests an important role for patients in improving decision quality. Furthermore, evidence suggests that patients can participate in such fateful treatment decisions and that their outcomes are better when they do. Two papers from England are particularly relevant for patients with breast cancer. The first demonstrates that nearly all women can make a choice when an effort is made to provide a balanced presentation of advantages and disadvantages of BCS and modified mastectomy. In this study, the majority of women chose mastectomy, most frequently citing concerns about risk of recurrence in the preserved breast and the possibility of completing primary therapy sooner.[43] The second study was designed to examine the relationship between therapy and psychosocial outcomes. It was found that whether or not women were given a choice was of greater relevance to those outcomes than the type of operation performed. Women who were provided a choice had better attitudes toward the future and better physical and psychological functioning.[37]

Additional evidence suggests that patients benefit from being involved in decision making. Patients with diabetes and ulcer disease who were coached to be more involved in treatment decisions had better functional status outcomes than counterparts.[38-40] However, the desire for involvement in decision making is not universal. Although being informed about treatment options and possible outcomes is highly valued by almost all patients, a significant number of patients would prefer to have their physician bear the responsibility of the treatment decision.[41-43] This preference may be explained by confusion on the part of patients about the nature of the decisions. Many patients fail to appreciate that the probabilities of outcomes vary systematically with different treatments and that the correct choice may depend as much on how patients value these different outcomes as on technical considerations. This distinction and the implications for doctors' and patients' decision-making roles is critical to decision-making quality.

If we assume that the man with coronary disease and the woman with breast cancer want to be involved in the treatment decision, what do they need in order to participate meaningfully in the decision process? As we as doctors try to improve the quality of decision making, how do we control sources of unwanted variation—variation that is a threat to quality—that may be associated with patient involvement in medical decision making?

Information Needs and Sources of Unwanted Variation in Decision Making

Clearly, one of the most important threats to quality of decision making when patients are involved is variation in the quality of information available to patients. Information needs of the patient involved in decision making are substantial. The patient must understand the full range of treatment options that are available. Further, he or she must understand the probability of good and bad outcomes that are contingent on each treatment choice. Finally, and perhaps most important, patients must have a basis for appreciating how different achievable outcomes will affect them personally—their quality of life, how they feel about themselves, and their ability to work and function from day to day.

Although patients may have alternative sources of such information, they rely heavily on their physicians. One can infer from the phenomenon of practice variation that the amount and content of information provided by different doctors is highly variable. One source of this variation is attitudinal. Some physicians are far less inclined to share information with patients, presumably on the basis of assessments of their wants and needs. Recommendations may be made without taking the time to share information or to sensitize patients to the role of their values in the treatment decision. The acceptance of such recommendations by poorly informed patients has been documented among women with early-stage breast cancer.[44] Results of second-opinion programs demonstrate the same dependence on physician judgment among many patients with ischemic heart disease.[45]

Another source of variation in the information presented by physicians to patients is professional uncertainty about the probabilities of outcomes. It is important to recognize different forms of professional uncertainty about treatments and their consequences. These forms of uncertainty can be thought of as sources of unwanted variation, each requiring a different approach to control. Because there is substantial variability in physicians' familiarity with evidence for or against clinical effectiveness of alternative treatments, one doctor may be uncertain about outcomes, whereas another is not. Alternatively, doctors who are equally familiar with the same data may interpret them differently and reach different conclusions. Often, however, clinical decisions must be made in the face of collective professional uncertainty; that is, no one can accurately estimate the probabilities because the research has not been done and the relevant evidence does not exist. Finally, no matter how much research has been done and how knowledgeable the clinician may be, the future can never be predicted with certainty. For example, even when the estimate of operative mortality is accurate and precise, irreducible stochastic uncertainty for any given patient remains. This information may be presented to patients differently by different physicians who have different attitudes toward these inherent risks.

Estimating Outcomes Probabilities: Where the Numbers Come From

A closer look at sources of professional knowledge will provide some insight about approaches to controlling sources of unwanted variation. For the man with ischemic heart disease, the choice between CABG, PTCA, or continued medical therapy depends on probability estimates. If the physician recommends CABG or PTCA, the most likely outcome will be symptom relief, but there is a chance of a complication with a serious result, even death. CABG, in particular, confers real risk of perioperative stroke or other neurological complications. There is also a chance that either procedure will fail to relieve symptoms or that any relief will be short-lived. If the physician recommends continued medical therapy, there is a chance that symptoms will improve, but it is more likely that the patient will continue to live with them. The risk of death in future years may be influenced also by the treatment choice.

The woman with breast cancer faces two sequential decisions: should she undergo BCS followed by radiation or mastectomy? Should she receive adjuvant therapy, either hormonal or cytotoxic? These decisions, too, depend on probabilities of good and bad outcomes. Where do these probabilities come from?

One source of these estimates is the doctor's collective past experience with patients similar to the patient at hand who underwent alternative treatments. This source constitutes the clinical experience so important to clinical judgment. For many conditions and treatments, the clinical experience of a single practitioner or group of practitioners is the primary source of probability estimates. But real problems are associated with this source of information. First, problems exist with the detail and accuracy with which clinicians characterize individual patients and thereby identify those who are similar to each other. Second, clinical practice is not standardized, and interventions are not carefully defined and uniformly applied. In addition, interventions evolve over time, with changes in surgical technique or in available pharmaceutical interventions. This evolution makes it difficult to attribute differences in outcome to a particular intervention. Third, there is no routine mechanism to define outcomes with the appropriate level of detail or to aggregate and organize the information that could be derived from collective clinical experience. Without such systematic aggregation and analysis, the cognitive heuristics that we all use routinely may mislead the clinician's unaided intuitive probability estimate. Sources of unwanted variation are evident here.

Recognizing these problems, those in the profession rely heavily on published clinical research—when it is available—to reduce professional uncertainty and thus reduce unwanted variation in the information supplied to patients. The randomized trial is the standard against which other clinical studies are measured. Information about patients entering the trial is collected systematically. The group is made homogeneous by applying exclusion and inclusion criteria. The alternative interventions are carefully defined and their elements carefully segregated. And outcomes—at least one or two of the more objective outcomes—are carefully catalogued. The scientific requirements of research designed to determine the effectiveness of one intervention relative to another, which is nothing more than the relative outcome probabilities, include similarity of the initial states, the integrity of the interventions, and similarity of detection or measurement of outcomes. Simply put, the methodological rigor of clinical trials is an attempt to standardize inputs, processes, and outcome measures to eliminate sources of variation that otherwise might confound inferences about the effectiveness of therapeutic interventions that are varied intentionally. Randomization is an effort to account for input (patient) variation that cannot otherwise be controlled.

As noted, clinical research that meets these requirements is the exception, rather than the rule. In the case of many common conditions and treatments, no randomized trials are available. Treatment of ischemic heart disease and breast cancer are such exceptions. CABG may be the most studied surgical procedure in history. Five randomized trials, including three large multicenter studies, compare CABG with medical therapy.[46-48] Trials comparing PTCA with medical therapy and CABG are just becoming available.[49-51] Hundreds of trials of surgical and adjuvant therapy have been conducted among women with early breast cancer.[27,28]

Even when well-conducted randomized trials are available, problems arise in using the results to estimate outcome probabilities. Clinicians may forget about real differences between the circumstances of the clinical trial and the circumstances of clinical practice. Effectiveness of interventions may be substantially different in the highly controlled, standardized "laboratory" environment of the trial than in actual practice. Clinicians also may forget about the patients excluded from the clinical trials. These exclusions are not trivial; in some cases, such as the CABG trials, the exclusions represent as many as 90 percent of the patients for whom the intervention would be used in practice.[52] The exclusions are important because different patients face different outcome probabilities even when the care rendered is identical. Any inference about the effectiveness of a particular intervention must adjust for different mixes of patients with different outcome probabilities. Generalization of trial results to excluded patients, often older or sicker, can result in inaccurate probability estimates for most patients.

Also, unwanted variation occurs in the way trial results are interpreted. Early interpretation of the CABG trials led many to the conclusion that CABG prolonged life for discrete subgroups of patients defined by coronary anatomy. Statistically significant survival differences were detected first among patients with disease of the left main coronary artery, then among those with three-vessel disease, and then among those with two-vessel disease and depressed cardiac function. Subsequently, on the strength of additional data, much of them derived from observational studies, it became clear that any survival advantage was due to a proportional reduction in baseline hazard of death. The size of the proportional reduction was a function of the coronary anatomy; the baseline risk was a function of the medical severity of the heart disease.[53] The discrete clinical groups identified early were those for which the proportional hazard reduction of a baseline risk resulted in a difference in absolute survival probability large enough to be identified by the power of the study.

Different clinical opinion leaders often find themselves at different places during the ongoing evolution of our understanding of treatment effectiveness. This variation among opinion leaders may reflect differences either in familiarity with data or methods of interpretation. Alternatively, clinical leaders may differ in their attitudes toward the risk of concluding incorrectly that a treatment is ineffective or effective. These differences in attitude often can be traced to different value judgments about the potential harms and benefits of treatment.

Analogous differences are found in interpretation of trial data for treatment of early breast cancer. Interpretation of initial trials of adjuvant therapy concluded that therapy was beneficial for discrete groups of patients, those at the highest risk of recurrence. It is now becoming clear that adjuvant therapy provides a similar proportional reduction in risk of recurrence and death to all women with early-stage breast cancer.[27,28] That proportional reduction was identified by early trials when, combined with a high baseline risk, it produced a large absolute difference in survival probabilities.

The trials that have had the greatest impact on our understanding of the relative effectiveness of BCS and mastectomy have been misinterpreted by many. When the NSABP 06 trial results were published, survival curves for each treatment were compared for overall survival, distant disease-free survival, and disease-free survival.[25,26] No differences were found between survival curves for BCS followed by radiation and mastectomy. The "disease-free" curves, however, did not include cancer recurrences in the breast retained by women treated with BCS. The report's authors reasoned that this finding would lead to misunderstanding because women who had mastectomy were not subject to such in-breast recurrences on the same side as the original cancer. This reasoning is presented clearly in the methods section of the papers. Furthermore, the authors later published the in-breast recurrence rates (approximately 1.5 percent per year) in a separate article.[54] Nevertheless, the presentation in the original papers led many to believe that no difference was found in overall recurrence rates, creating an unwanted source of variation in the information presented to women at the time of a treatment decision.

Availability of data from clinical trials, applicability of the data to the patient at hand and to interventions available, and correct interpretation of the data are all important to decision quality. But even when these criteria are met, there is a need to be vigilant about the currency of information. Consider the advances that have been made in the treatment of coronary disease since the

TABLE 4.2 Threats to Decision Quality: Professional Uncertainty

Information does not exist/relevant research has not been done
Information does exist but is inaccessible
To clinicians in general
To particular clinician(s)
Information accessible but subject to variable interpretation
Variable professional response to irreducible uncertainty

major randomized trials were conducted. New medical therapeutics have been introduced. Surgical technique has been advanced dramatically by cold cardioplegia and use of artery implants, as well as by vein grafts. Angioplasty arrived on the scene. Similar advances in breast cancer care have occurred. A strong argument can be made for making outcomes research among intelligently sampled subsets of patients a routine part of clinical care. Such an approach to continuously improving the knowledge base as technology advances would not substitute for randomized trials, but would be a very valuable additional source of information to support decision quality.

Threats to decision quality related to professional knowledge are summarized in Table 4.2.

Values and Preferences: Controlling Variation or Celebrating It?

Outcomes research has the potential to dramatically improve the clinician's ability to accurately estimate clinically relevant outcome probabilities. These probabilities are necessary but not sufficient to ensure decision quality. Each person with ischemic heart disease and each woman with breast cancer is unique. Clinical trials and outcomes research focus on homogeneous subsets of patients to better isolate the effects of treatment on outcome and to make ever more accurate and precise estimates of outcome probabilities. But heterogeneity within these groups is inevitable. Different patients have different subjective responses to the same outcomes. They have different attitudes toward the same degree of risk. And some are more willing than others to incur risk or morbidity now for some putative future benefit. When considering decision quality, these sources of variation are not unwanted. To the extent that they define the uniqueness of the individual patient, they are critical determinants of "the right thing to do" for that patient.

For the patient with ischemic heart disease, the decision to perform CABG depends heavily on judgments about the impact of symptoms on the quality of life. The benefit of symptom relief must be weighed against the harms associated with stroke, cognitive dysfunction, and other possible complications of surgery. Different men and women apply different weights. For many with coronary disease, risk of death is reduced by CABG. But to achieve the survival benefit, one first must accept the risk of operative mortality, which increases substantially the relative risk of death over the short term. Different patients have very different levels of acceptable risk and make different trade-offs over time.

Similar value judgments are central to decisions about breast cancer treatment. When choosing between BCS and radiation and mastectomy, quality-of-life considerations dominate. Survival is equivalent with either approach. The woman's decision hinges on how she feels about keeping her breast and the attendant marginal increase in risk of having to deal with breast cancer again because of a recurrence in that breast. The adjuvant therapy decision is equally value dependent. Most women with early breast cancer are cured by BCS and radiation or mastectomy, but all women face some risk of recurrence that varies, depending on certain clinical characteristics. Adjuvant therapy can reduce that risk by about 30 percent, producing what may seem like a substantial absolute risk reduction for the woman at high baseline risk. But that benefit decreases for the woman at low risk, and the treatment often exacts a heavy toll, conferring significant morbidity for six months with some side effects, such as premature menopause, that are permanent. As with ischemic heart disease, the right decision depends on weights assigned by unique patients to the good and bad outcomes, the level of risk reduction that justifies the short- and long-term morbidity, and the time trade-offs.

How confident can a patient be about making the value judgments concerned with health outcomes that can be such important determinants of treatment choice? The patient may have more confidence in making a determination about the quality of life impact of a state that he or she has experienced than one that must be imagined. Such imaginings may be helped by the vicarious experience of other patients who have been in the unfamiliar state. Physicians can provide such vicarious experience, but it severely tests their communication skills. Variability in physicians' effectiveness in dealing with these communication tasks is another important source of variation in the decision-making process. The patient may not be educated about the role of values and preferences in making the right treatment choice. The physician may fail to effectively elicit preferences or may make incorrect inferences about what the patient values on the basis of his or her own preferences. Few resources are available to clinicians to support this role. Systematically collected data documenting patients' subjective responses to illness and treatment are scarce.

Outcomes research could provide a database that would generate not only information about outcome probabilities but also a context for value judgments. In developing such a database, researchers could test available methods for the assessment of values or preferences. Preferences for the same health states vary not only among patients but also over time for the same patient. Preferences are influenced easily by the context of the decision or the measurement task used. But further work in this area could reduce unwanted variation in the communication and perception of the subjective elements of health care decisions. It also could provide measures of patients' preferences that could be used to assess decision quality.[55,56]

Model for Improvement of Performance and Decision Quality

The potential for a synthesis of IQMS and outcomes research to improve quality of performance and decision making may be made clear by describing a system that achieves this synthesis. The requirements for such a system are displayed schematically in Figure 4.1. The system must first capture patient characteristics that are likely to affect outcomes. These characteristics—especially disease severity and comorbidity—must be controlled for in attributing outcomes to treatments. The techniques of IQMS then can be used in real time and retrospectively to characterize the processes of care, to identify sources of variability in those processes, to relate variability in processes to variability in outcomes, and to provide guidance on how to improve performance quality. Patients' perceptions of some aspects of the process of care may be useful in monitoring performance and may assist providers to better understand and respond to variations in the execution of treatment plans.

Outcome measures, preferably focusing on those outcomes most important to patients, are another essential element. These include patient reports of symptom status and other subjective variables. Outcome measures also should include patients' ratings of health states and the effects of those states on quality of life.

The logistics of such a system are not simple. Perhaps the most difficult task is assembling clinically coherent and distinct cohorts of patients. Ideally, the system would collect patient descriptors before treatment decisions are made so as to minimize the possible biases that treatment choice may create in subsequent data collection. With standardized measures of baseline severity and comorbidity, process, and outcomes, large databases could be developed that would improve estimates of probability of outcome for many common conditions and treatments. Standardized measures also would make possible clinically credible comparisons of outcomes achieved by different providers using the same intervention. Linked to measures of process, which are likely to vary significantly among

FIGURE 4.1 Collective Experience as a Source of New Knowledge

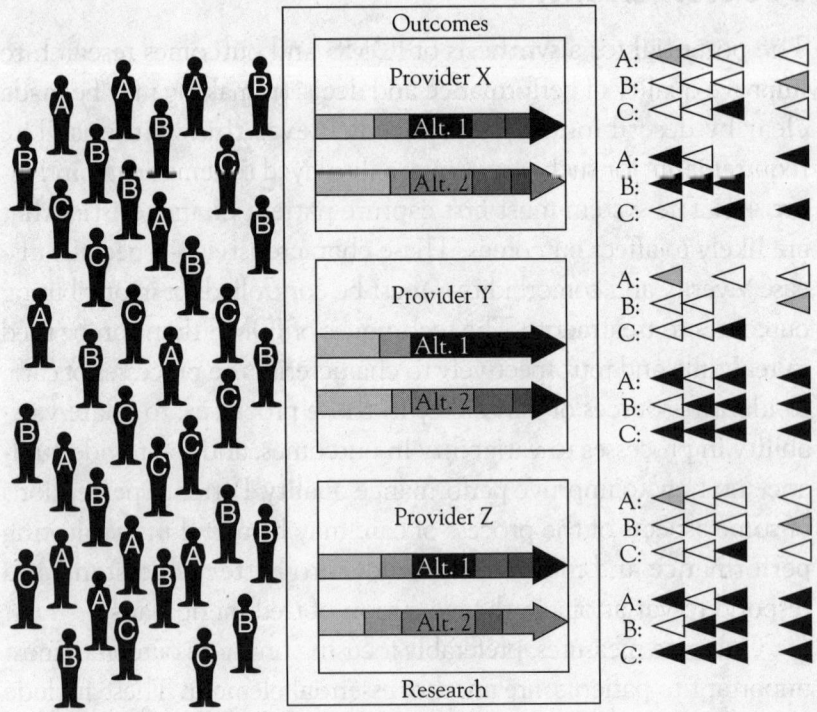

Figure 4.1 is a model for synthesizing IQMS and outcomes research indicating the required data on patient characteristics, processes of care, and outcomes. The stick figures represent patients, each labeled A, B, or C. Each has different clinical characteristics that might influence outcomes. The pairs of arrows indicate alternative treatments that might be rendered by different providers, labeled X, Y, and Z. Note that different providers use different proportions of the same inputs or elements of care process in delivering the same treatment interventions as indicated by the different patterns within arrows. The triangles represent different achievable outcomes following treatment. The synthesis of IQMS and outcomes research requires (1) measures of patient characteristics, including disease severity and comorbidity, (2) measures of process as care is delivered by different providers, and (3) measures of outcomes. Patients' reports of process and outcomes supplement other sources of information. For some outcomes, they represent the only valid source of information. Patient ratings of process (satisfaction with care) and outcomes (utility or well-being for different health states) are necessary to ensure that care is patient centered and that decisions reflect patients' values and preferences.

providers, these outcome comparisons would provide the gist for true benchmarking and improvement in process design and performance.

The development of process measures and their correlation with outcomes is essential to improving performance quality. The development of outcome data and the correlation of such outcomes with treatment decisions are essential to improving decision quality. In the latter case, the collective experience of past patients must be fed back to help current decision making. A good example of this potential is the Duke Cardiovascular Databank, which includes the experience of nearly twenty thousand patients treated with either medical therapy, CABG, or PTCA. Statistical models derived from their outcome experience can provide, for patients with very specific clinical characteristics, accurate probability estimates of symptom relief and survival following any one of these treatment choices. These estimates, complemented by other information, including that derived from randomized trials, can be generated easily by computers and presented to doctor and patient in a standardized, understandable format.

Interactive videodisc programs have been developed to assist doctors and patients in these tasks. Such programs use extensive interviews with patients and clinicians during design and evaluation to assure that presentations are accurate and balanced. These shared decision-making programs reduce unwanted variation in the information provided patients as part of the decision process, thereby improving decision quality.[55-57]

Another type of feedback can help patients appreciate and allow for the role of their personal values and preferences in decision making, thereby improving decision quality. The experience of previous patients who already have made treatment choices and experienced different outcomes can be made available to current patients. Previous patients' descriptions of their experiences can help new patients imagine what life will be like with different outcomes. This element of shared decision-making programs has been highly valued by patients facing difficult choices.

These two feedback loops, continuously improving the professional knowledge about which interventions work for whom and continuously improving our understanding of what is valued by those who live with the consequences of decisions, are displayed in Figure 4.2.[18]

FIGURE 4.2 Information Flow for Continuous Improvement of Decision Quality and Performance Quality

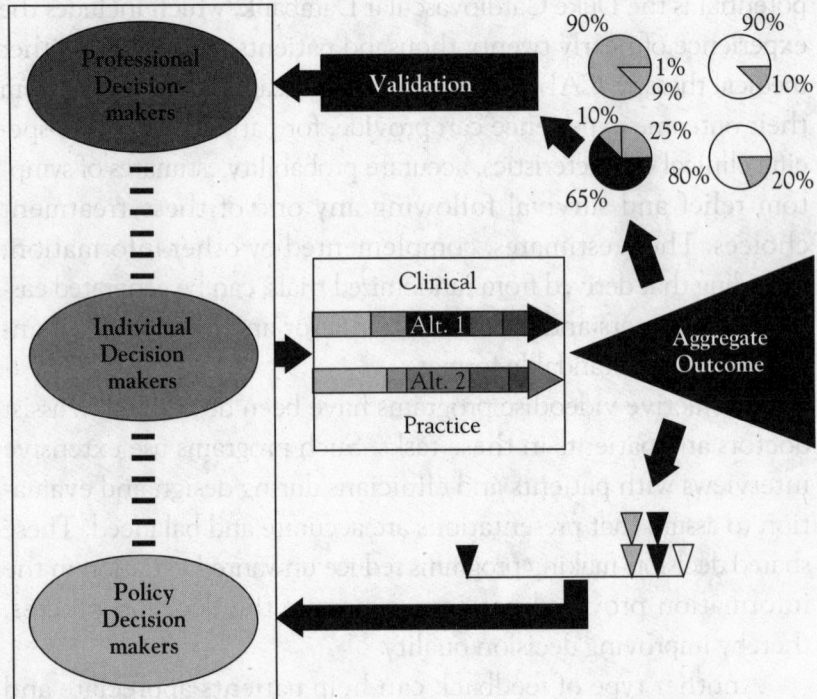

Two feedback loops support and continuously improve decision quality. The pie diagrams along the upper loop represent (1) outcome probability estimates for different treatments and (2) comparative outcome rates for different providers using the same interventions. Calculated patient-specific probability estimates can inform individual decisions. The comparative rates can stimulate examination and improvement of processes. The linear scales along the lower loop represent patients' individual and aggregate subjective responses to achievable health outcomes, which are represented by the triangles. This flow of "vicarious experience" can help sensitize patients to the importance of their personal values in decision making. Patients' responses to health outcomes also can serve to inform policy judgments about the value of alternative investments in health care.

Treatment outcomes of breast cancer and ischemic heart disease are two of many clinical situations in which shared decision-making programs—which synthesize IQMs and outcomes research—could reduce undesirable practice variation by supporting the doctor and the patient in the communication tasks necessary to make the right choice for each patient. If two patient populations had the same distributions of preferences (including attitudes toward risks and trade-offs over time), the sum of informed individual choices would produce the same use rates among those populations. In contrast, with the use of guidelines or critical paths to standardize care comes the risk of imposing standardized preferences on all patients, prescribing interventions to some patients who would not choose them and withholding interventions from some who would.

The model described here, with its focus on improving quality in the decision-making process and recognizing the roles and responsibilities of doctors and patients, would achieve reduction in unwanted and undesirable practice variation by respecting the prerogatives and uniqueness of those who live with the decisions and outcomes. As medical professionals struggle to redefine their role in a changing health care economy, the tools derived from IQMS and outcomes research will be essential in efforts to become more accountable for keeping and advancing a knowledge base and for using that knowledge to meet the needs of patients and society.

Notes

1. Luft, H. S., Bunker, J. P., & Enthoven, A. C. (1979). Should operations be regionalized? *New England Journal of Medicine, 301,* 1364–1369.

2. Showstack, J. A., Rosenfeld, K. E., Garnick, D. W., Luft, H. S., Schaffarzick, R. W., & Fowles, J. (1987). Association of volume with outcome of coronary artery bypass graft surgery. *Journal of the American Medical Association, 257,* 785–789.

3. Hannan, E. L., O'Donnell, J. F., Kilburn, H., Bernard, H. R., & Yazici, A. (1989). Investigation of the relationship between volume and mortality for surgical procedures performed in New York State hospitals. *Journal of the American Medical Association, 262,* 503–510.

4. Health Care Financing Administration. (1987). *Medicare hospital mortality information—1986.* Washington, DC: Author.

5. Wennberg, J., & Gittelsohn, A. (1973). Small area variations in health care delivery. *Science, 182,* 1102–1108.

6. Wennberg, J. E., & Gittelsohn, A. (1982). Variations in medical care among small areas. *Scientific American, 246,* 120–134.

7. Chassin, M. R., Brook, R. H., Park, R. E., Keesey, J., Fink, A., Kosecoff, J., Kahn, K., Merrick, N., & Solomon, D. H. (1986). Variations in the use of medical and surgical services by the Medicare population. *New England Journal of Medicine, 314,* 285–90.

8. Chassin, M. R., Kosecoff, J., Park, R. E., Winslow, C. M., Kahn, K. L., Merrick, N. J., Keesey, J., Fink, A., Solomon, D. H., & Brook, R. H. (1987). Does inappropriate use explain geographic variations in the use of health care services? *Journal of the American Medical Association, 258,* 2533–2537.

9. Bunker, J. P. (1990). Variations in hospital admissions and the appropriateness of care: American preoccupations? *British Medical Journal, 301*(6751), 531–532.

10. Wenneker, M. B., & Epstein, A. M. (1989). Racial inequalities in the use of procedures for patients with ischemic heart disease in Massachusetts. *Journal of the American Medical Association, 26*(2), 253–257.

11. Greenfield, S., Blanco, D. M., Elashoff, R. M., & Ganz, P. A. (1987). Patterns of care related to age of breast cancer patients. *Journal of the American Medical Association, 257,* 2766–2770.

12. Held, P. J., Pauly, M. V., Boubjerg, J. D., Newmann, J., & Salvateira, O., Jr. (1988). Access to kidney transplantation: Has the United States eliminated income and racial differences? *Archives of Internal Medicine, 148,* 2594–2600.

13. Lohr, K. N. (Ed.). (1990). *Medicare: A strategy for quality assurance* (Vol. 1). Washington, DC: National Academy Press.

14. American College of Cardiology. (1993). Guidelines for percuta-
    neous transluminal coronary angioplasty. *Journal of the American
    College of Cardiology, 22,* 2033–2054.

15. New York State Department of Health. (1993). *Coronary artery
    bypass surgery in New York State 1990–1992.* Albany: Author.

16. Wennberg, J. E., Freeman, J. L., & Culp, W. J. (1987). Are hospital
    services rationed in New Haven or over-utilised in Boston? *Lancet,
    1,* 1185–1189.

17. American College of Cardiology. (1991). Guidelines and indica-
    tions for coronary artery bypass graft surgery. *Circulation, 83,*
    1125–1172.

18. Leape, L. L., Hilborne, L. H., Kahan, J. P., et al. (1991). *Coronary
    artery bypass graft: A literature review and ratings of appropriateness
    and necessity.* Santa Monica, CA: RAND.

19. Hilborne, L. H., Leape, L. L., Kahan, J. P., et al. (1991). *Percuta-
    neous transluminal coronary angioplasty: A literature review and ratings
    of appropriateness and necessity.* Santa Monica, CA: RAND.

20. Mulley, A. G., & Eagle, K. A. (1988). What is inappropriate care?
    Journal of the American Medical Association, 260, 540–541.

21. Doliszny, K. M., Luepker, R. V., Burke, G. L., Pryor, D. B., Black-
    burn, H. (1994). Estimated contribution of coronary artery bypass
    graft surgery to the decline in coronary heart disease mortality. The
    Minnesota heart survey. *Journal of the American College of Cardiol-
    ogy, 24*(1), 95–103.

22. Harris, J. R., Lippman, M. E., Veronesi, U., & Willett, W. (1992).
    Breast cancer: Part I. *New England Journal of Medicine, 327*(5),
    319–328.

23. Veronesi, U., Saccozzi, R., Del Vecchio, M., Banfi, A., Clemente,
    C., De Lena, M., Gallus, G., Greco, M., Luini, A., Marubini, E.,
    Muscolinio, G., Rilke, F., Salvadori, B., Zecchini, A., & Zucali, R.
    (1981). Comparing radical mastectomy with quadrantectomy, axil-
    lary dissection, and radiotherapy in patients with small cancers of
    the breast. *New England Journal of Medicine, 305*(1), 6–11.

24. Veronesi, U., Banfi, A., Salvadori, B., et al. (1990). Breast conserva-
    tion is the treatment of choice in small breast cancer: Long-term
    results of a randomized trial. *European Journal of Cancer, 26,* 668–670.

25. Fisher, B., Bauer, M., Margolese, R., Poisson, R., Pilch, Y., Redmond, C., Fisher, E., Wolmark, N., Deutsch, M., Montague, E., Saffer, E., Wickerham, L., Lerner, H., Glass, A., Shibata, H., Deckers, P., Ketcham, A., Oishi, R., & Russell, I. (1985). Five-year results of a randomized clinical trial comparing total mastectomy and segmental mastectomy with or without radiation in the treatment of breast cancer. *New England Journal of Medicine, 312*(11), 665–673.

26. Fisher, B., Redmond, C., Poisson, R., Margolese, R., Wolmark, N., Wickerham, L., Fisher, E., Deutsch, M., Caplan, R., Pilch, Y., Glass, A., Shibata, H., Lerner, H., Terz, J., & Sidorovich, L. (1989). Eight-year results of a randomized clinical trial comparing total mastectomy and lumpectomy with or without irradiation in the treatment of breast cancer. *New England Journal of Medicine, 320,* 822–828.

27. Early Breast Cancer Trialists' Collaborative Group. (1988). Effects of adjuvant tamoxifen and cytotoxic therapy on mortality in early breast cancer. *New England Journal of Medicine, 319,* 1681–1692.

28. Early Breast Cancer Trialists' Collaborative Group. (1992). Systemic treatment of early breast cancer by hormonal, cytotoxic, or immune therapy. *Lancet, 339,* 1–15, 71–85.

29. Farrow, D. C., Hunt, W. C., & Samet, J. M. (1992). Geographic variation in the treatment of localized breast cancer. *New England Journal of Medicine, 326*(17), 1097–1101.

30. Nattinger, A. B., Gottlieb, M. S., Veum, J., Yahnke, D., & Goodwin, J. S. (1992). Geographic variation in the use of breast-conserving treatment for breast cancer. *New England Journal of Medicine, 326*(17), 1102–1107.

31. NIH Consensus Conference Statement. (1980). Adjuvant chemotherapy for breast cancer. *New England Journal of Medicine, 303,* 830–832.

32. NIH Consensus Conference Statement. (1985). Adjuvant chemotherapy for breast cancer. *Journal of the American Medical Association, 254,* 3461–3463.

33. NIH Consensus Conference. (1991). Treatment of early-stage breast cancer. *Journal of the American Medical Association, 265,* 391–395.

34. Tarbox, B., Rockwood, J., & Abernathy, C. (1992). Are modified radical mastectomies done for T1 breast cancer because of surgeon's advice or patient's choice? *American Journal of Surgery, 164,* 417–422.

35. GIVIO (Interdisciplinary Group for Cancer Care Evaluation). (1988). Survey of treatment of primary breast cancer in Italy. *British Journal of Cancer, 57,* 630–634.

36. Wilson, R. G., Hart, A., & Dawes, P.J.D.K. (1988). Mastectomy or conservation: The patient's choice. *British Medical Journal, 297*(6657), 1167–1169.

37. Morris, T., & Ingham, R. (1988). Choice of surgery for early breast cancer: Psychosocial considerations. *Social Science and Medicine, 27,* 1257–1262.

38. Greenfield, S., Kaplan, S., & Ware, J. (1985). Expanding patient involvement in care: Effects on patient outcomes. *Annals of Internal Medicine, 102,* 520–528.

39. Greenfield, S., Kaplan, S. H., Ware, J. E., Yano, E. M., & Frank, H. J. (1988). Patients' participation in medical care: Effects on blood sugar control and quality of life in diabetes. *Journal of General Medicine, 3,* 448.

40. Kaplan, S. H., Greenfield, S., & Ware, J. (1989). Assessing the effects of physician-patient interactions on the outcomes of chronic disease. *Medical Care, 27,* S110–S127.

41. Brody, D. S. (1980). The patients' role in clinical decision making. *Annals of Internal Medicine, 93,* 718–722.

42. Strull, W. B., Lo, B., & Charles, G. (1984). Do patients want to participate in medical decision making? *Journal of the American Medical Association, 252,* 2990–2994.

43. Ende, J., Kazis, L., Ash, A., & Moskowitz, M. A. (1989). Measuring patients' desire for autonomy: Decision making and information seeking preferences among medical patients. *Journal of General Internal Medicine, 4,* 23–33.

44. Siminoff, L. A., & Fetting, J. H. (1991). Factors affecting treatment decisions for a life-threatening illness: The case of medical treatment of breast cancer. *Social Science and Medicine, 32*(7), 813–818.

45. Graboys, T. B., Headly, A., Lown, B., Lampert, S., & Blatt, C. M. (1987). Results of a second opinion program for coronary artery bypass graft surgery. *Journal of the American Medical Association, 258,* 1611–1614.

46. Veterans Administration Coronary Artery Bypass Surgery Cooperative Study Group. (1984). Eleven-year survival in the Veterans Administration randomized trail of coronary bypass surgery for stable angina. *New England Journal of Medicine, 311,* 1333–1339.

47. European Coronary Surgery Study Group. (1982). Long-term results of prospective randomized study of coronary bypass surgery for stable angina pectoris. *Lancet, 2,* 1173–1180.

48. CASS Principal Investigators. (1984). Myocardial infarction and survival in the CASS randomized trial. *New England Journal of Medicine, 310,* 750–758.

49. BARI, CABRI, EAST, GABI, and RITA. (1990). Coronary angioplasty on trial. *Lancet, 335,* 1315–1316.

50. Parisi, A. F., Folland, E. D., Hartigan, P., et al. (1992). A comparison of angioplasty with medical therapy in the treatment of single-vessel coronary artery disease. *New England Journal of Medicine, 326,* 10–16.

51. RITA Trial Participants. (1993). Coronary angioplasty versus coronary artery bypass surgery: The Randomised Intervention Treatment of Angina trial. *Lancet, 341,* 573–580.

52. Hlatky, M. A., Califf, R. M., Harrell, F. E., Lee, K. L., Mark, D. B., & Pryor, D. B. (1988). Comparison of predictions based on observational data with the results of randomized controlled clinical trials of coronary bypass surgery. *Journal of the American College of Cardiology, 11,* 237–245.

53. Califf, R. M., Harrell, F. E., Lee, K. L., et al. (1989). The evolution of medical and surgical therapy for coronary artery disease. *Journal of the American Medical Association, 261,* 2077–2086.

54. Fisher, B., Anderson, S., Fisher, E. R., Redmond, C., Wickerham, D. L., Wolmark, N., Mamounas, E. P., Deutsch, M., & Margolese, R. (1991). Significance of ipsilateral breast tumour recurrence after lumpectomy. *Lancet, 338,* 327–331.

55. Mulley, A. G. (1989). Assessing patients' utilities: Can the ends justify the means? *Medical Care, 27,* S269–S281.

56. Mulley, A. G. (1990). Medical decision making and practice variation. In T. F. Anderson & G. Mooney (Eds.), *The challenges of medical practice variations* (pp. 59–75). New York: Macmillan.

57. Kasper, J. F., Mulley, A. G., Jr., & Wennberg, J. E. (1992). Developing shared decision-making programs to improve the quality of health care. *Quality Review Bulletin,* pp. 183–190.

58. Mulley, A. G. (1990). Applying effectiveness and outcomes research to clinical practice. In K. A. Heithoff & K. N. Lohr (Eds.), *Effectiveness and outcomes in health care* (pp. 179–189). Washington, DC: National Academy Press.

PART TWO

Applications

5

Applying the Statistical Methods of Continuous Quality Improvement to Primary Care

Hypertension

Duncan Neuhauser, Ph.D., Linda Headrick, M.D., William Katcher, and Paulette Lucas

FACULTY: How could care be improved?

STUDENT: By having smarter patients.

The three Magic Valley Medical Center, Twin Falls, Idaho, questions:

Why do we do what we do?

How do we know it works?

What can we do to make it better?

What is good care for a person with hypertension? With asthma? With multiple sclerosis? How would you know good care if you saw it? These obvious questions deserve answers.

In struggling to answer these questions, we have come to accept a number of ideas based on the application of principles of continuous quality improvement (CQI) to clinical care:

1. *Patients are partners in their care, rather than passive customers.* This is rather obvious but all too rarely acted on. The ethos of medicine more often presents the expert physician and the passive, unknowing patient.

2. *A reasonably good working definition of good care is "the patient controlling the disease, rather than the disease controlling the patient."* This definition of self-mastery seems appropriate to such chronic conditions as asthma, hypertension, and diabetes. Another definition is "reduction of the burden of illness."

3. *To develop self-mastery of chronic disease, patients must have accurate mental models of their own conditions.* These models potentiate patients' understanding and controlling their diseases. A mental model is a set of ideas about how the world works—in this case, how the disease works—that assists in predicting the consequences of actions. "Exercise is more likely to give me an asthma attack when it is cold out, but being around cats does not bother me." This model has four variables—exercise, asthma, temperature, and cat dander—a dependent variable (asthma), and an interaction effect between exercise and temperature.

In this chapter, we show how one patient was helped to build such a model for her hypertension, made it quantitative and explicit, tested its accuracy, and shared it with her physician.

4. *Costs of care are important for the payer/customer/partner.* Our vision for good care is that it should be possible to improve quality at half the current cost.

5. *Physician incentives should not be based on fee-for-service income.* Instead, physicians should be rewarded for creating self-mastery for the patient. One is struck with how deeply ingrained fee-for-service thinking is in medical practice. Requiring regular return visits has become customary, rather than helping patients build self-management skills and thereby define the spacing of future visits. Health care reform, combined with CQI, may provide a great opportunity to rethink and modify the incentives that govern physician behavior.

6. *The physician can help the patient develop a mental model of his or her condition and learn how to reduce variation in his or her care, but it is ultimately up to the patient to comply with care recommendations.*

To evaluate the physician on the basis of compliance rates of her or his hypertensive patients is to assume that all power resides with the physician. Using such measures to judge physicians reflects the assumption of physician dominance, rather than of a partnership between patient and physician. Mellins and coauthors observed that patients "dump" 40 to 50 percent of what physicians prescribe, at least in part because they are not part of the decision-making process.[1]

7. *CQI posits two types of knowledge: professional knowledge and knowledge for improvement.* In medicine, *professional knowledge* focuses on pathophysiology and therapeutics. *Knowledge for improvement* includes systems thinking, understanding variation, and learning the psychology of motivation and theories of knowledge. A working hypothesis is that more than half of the variation in outcomes and costs of care is attributable to variables best understood through knowledge for improvement. This conclusion comes from analyzing variation in asthma care, costs, and outcomes over five years and hundreds of cases followed by medical students in Cleveland.[2-6] Variation often is due to failures of motivation and compliance; deficiencies in patient knowledge, such as inability to use inhalers correctly; and delivery system failures. These causes of variation are reported more frequently than explanations due to illness severity or differences in therapeutic effectiveness. Most medical education is focused on professional knowledge. A balanced combination of both types of knowledge makes better sense.

The seven concepts outlined above are summarized in Table 5.1. Our example of care for patients with high blood pressure reflects these ideas.

Two disease models are especially conducive to partnership thinking. One is diabetes, for which a substantial portion of care is self-managed. Greenfield, Kaplan, and coworkers demonstrated that diabetic patients encouraged to negotiate medical decisions with the doctor had improved glucose control and decreased func-

TABLE 5.1 Applying Principles of CQI to Medical Practice

Often observed now	More needed
Doctor knows best	Doctors and patients are partners
One physician/one patient working in isolation	Systems of care support the work of the patient-provider partnership
Doctor responsible for diagnosis and treatment	Doctor and patient share responsibility for patient self-mastery
Clinical judgment	Statistical-mindedness, understanding variation in support of clinical judgment
Costs do not matter	Costs matter
Short-term focus on each visit in a fee-for-service context	Care over time to manage costs over time
Episodic care of acute illness	Continuous care of chronic conditions
Doctor is held accountable for patient's compliance	Patient as partner has a major responsibility for compliance
Professional knowledge (exclusively the biomedical paradigm)	Professional knowledge and knowledge for improvement combined

tional limitations, with no loss of efficiency in the physician visit.[7] The second is AIDS, about which many patients are so knowledgeable that they challenge even those physicians who specialize in caring for such patients.

Here, hypertension is chosen for application of the principles of CQI. It seemed obvious to us that blood pressure is a process that could be tracked by using run charts. That is where our approach started.

As part of a pilot longitudinal learning project for medical students, five patients with high blood pressure were recruited at a county hospital. Four were assigned to students; one was followed by a faculty member (L.H.). The goal was for each student-patient pair to work as a team to study the process of antihypertensive care for that individual patient, to examine pertinent outcomes, and to use that knowledge to improve the patient's care. The initial task was to go through the patient's records and create a blood pressure run chart. In principle, the same exercise could be used for all patients, not just the five discussed here.

We believed we could find patients who would regularly monitor their blood pressures and participate in their own care. A number of studies have shown the benefit of home blood pressure monitoring for a variety of patient groups.[8-10] We know of no studies in which patients have participated in statistical analysis of the data, even with a simple run chart. A more relevant question is what percentage of hypertensive patients could and would do so? A convenience sample of five is better than one, but it is surely only a start to finding out how widespread such participation could be. Patients cared for in a county hospital system seem particularly appropriate for such a project because they might seem less likely to participate than highly educated patients from a suburban private practice.

Table 5.2 provides some descriptive information about the patients followed in the study reported here.

Hypertension Run Charts

Figure 5.1 shows a run chart for systolic and diastolic blood pressure for Patient A from September 1989 to February 1993, showing relatively little fluctuation—a stable process. Figure 5.2 shows systolic pressure from 1988 through 1992 for Patient D. For this patient, the fluctuations are greater. The medical student dug into the record and found that these variations were explained partly by multiple changes in medications. Immediately recalibrating treatment on the basis of blood pressure reading of the moment is the very opposite of CQI statistical thinking for stable processes. Later, the patient confided to the student that she often skipped her diuretic because of urinary frequency, perhaps also contributing to the observed fluctuations. Perhaps both examples shown in Figures 5.1 and 5.2 are found frequently in the practice of medicine.

TABLE 5.2 Five Hypertensive Patients (1992–1993)

Patient	Age	Gender	Run chart from record	Self-measurement
A	61	F	Y	N
B	71	F	Y	N
C	48	M	Y	N
D	68	F	Y	Y
E	48	F	Y	Y

Patient A: The patient was more concerned about her diabetes control than her hypertension. The student described her as having an "I will take a pill" approach to her hypertension. Costs of care were also an issue for this patient. Therefore, the patient was unwilling to keep routine follow-up appointments.

Patient B: Financial issues were also important in the care of this patient. The patient's previous physician provided free medication from drug detail samples. Her new physician was unable to do so. Confronted with $80-$90 each month for medication on an income of $400 per month, she often took less than prescribed or skipped the medicine altogether. At the urging of the medical student, the physician arranged a social work consultation and agreed to write to the drug company to ask for the medication at a reduced price.

Patient C: The patient expressed great interest in working with the student but missed many appointments. He expressed a desire to emphasize nonpharmacological therapy and to minimize his medications. He admitted that he often missed appointments when he was unable to carry out his plans to lose weight and exercise.

Patient D: The patient already had purchased a home blood pressure monitor. She was encouraged to record her readings. She brought these readings to her visits, and her providers used them to guide her therapy.

Patient E: This is the faculty member's patient described in text. The home blood pressure monitor was purchased by the physician.

Note: For the first four patients, variance in care because of costs, compliance, system changes, and lifestyle played important roles. In these areas, knowledge for improvement is relevant.

Patient E was invited to participate because of difficulty achieving good blood pressure control. She had tried multiple medication regimens but had experienced numerous side effects: edema with nifedipine, rash with an angiotensin-converting enzyme (ACE) inhibitor, and fatigue with a beta-blocker. After multiple adjustments, her diastolic blood pressure at office visits was still 100–110 on three medications: verapamil, clonidine, and hydrochlorothiazide (five pills per day).

FIGURE 5.1 Patient A: Run Chart of Systolic and Diastolic Blood Pressure Measurements

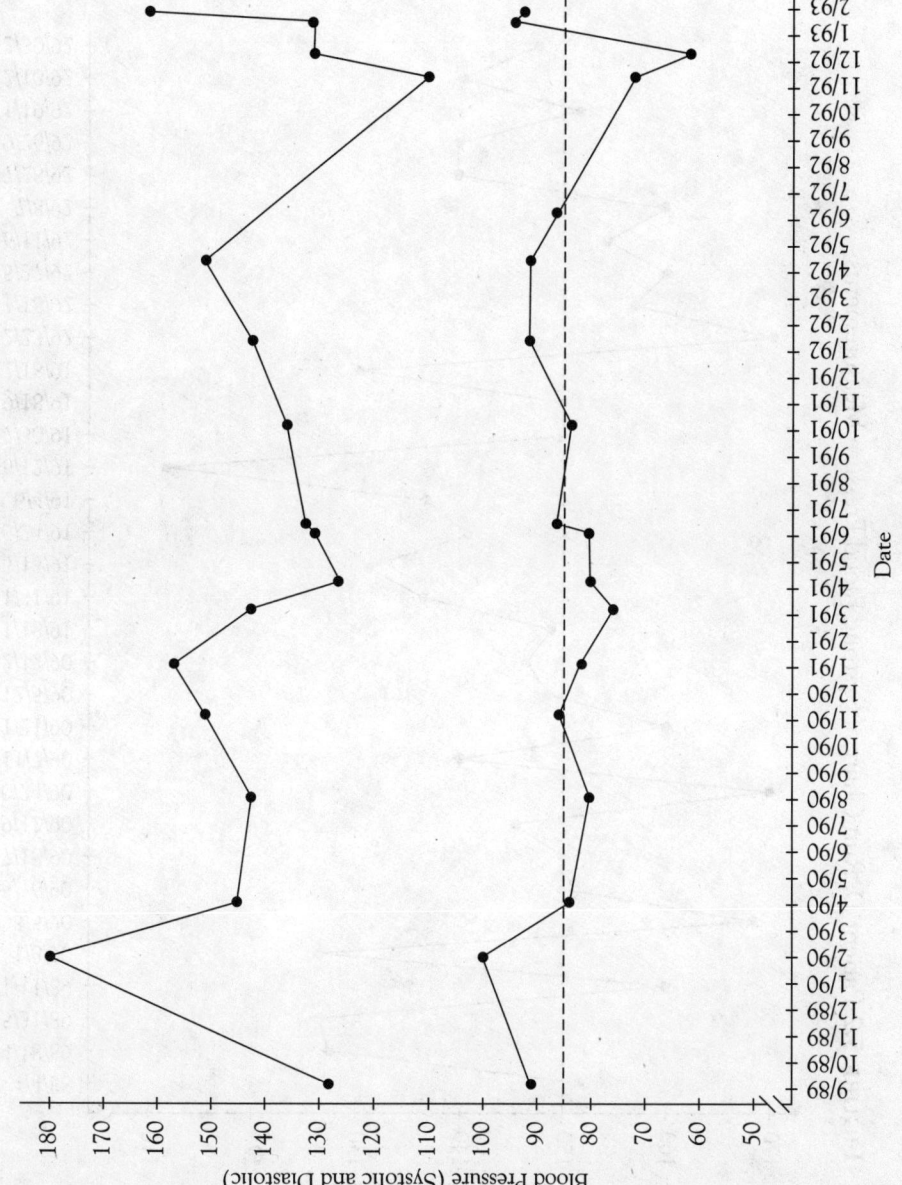

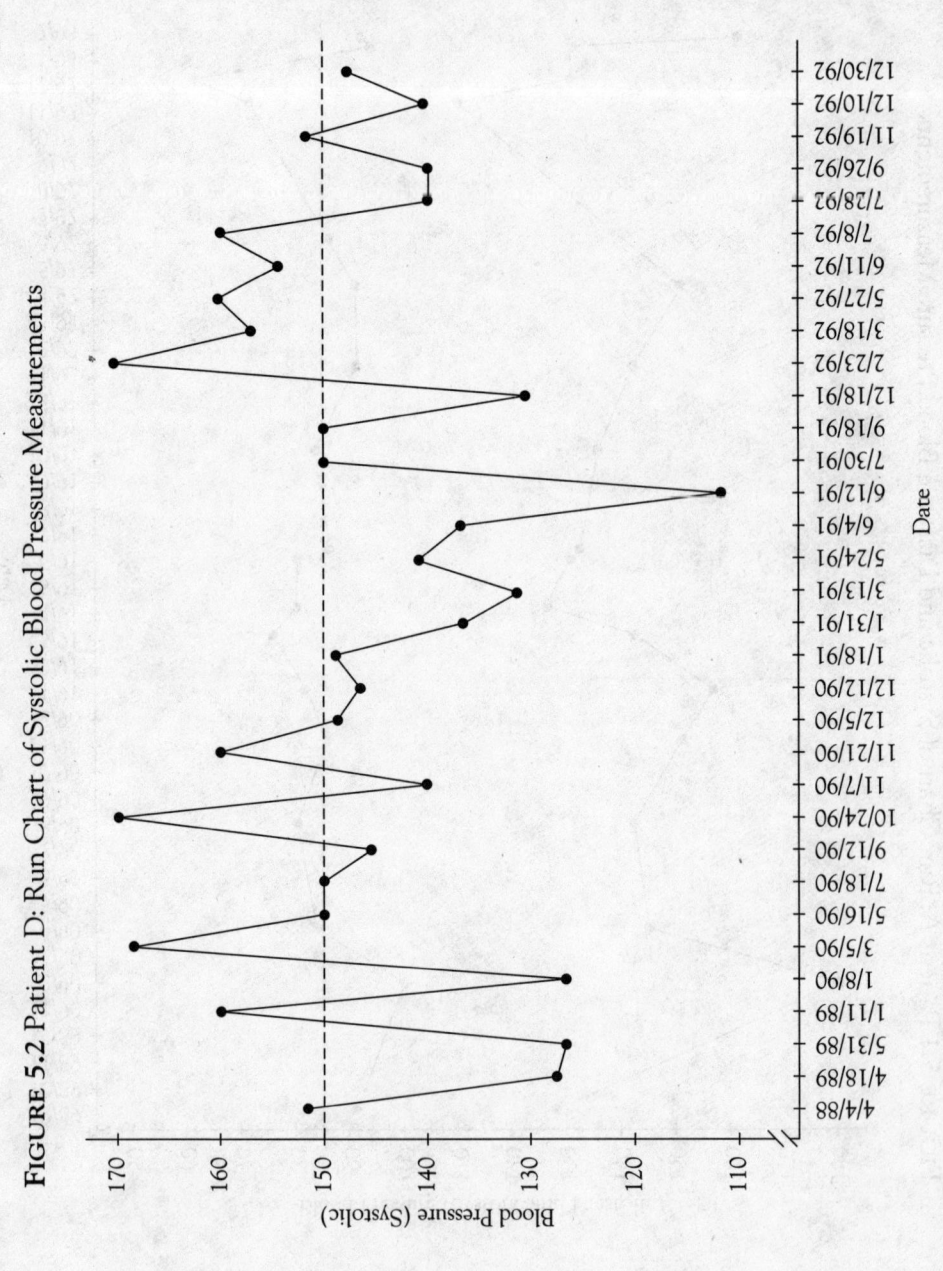

FIGURE 5.2 Patient D: Run Chart of Systolic Blood Pressure Measurements

Patient E and her physician sensed that "white coat hypertension" might be an issue, so she was encouraged to have her blood pressure checked elsewhere. She found it convenient to stop by a clinic near her home after work, usually at about 5 or 6 P.M. These readings were still in the 90–100 mm Hg range for diastolic blood pressure. On a few occasions when the pressure was higher, the patient panicked and called the physician, worried that a diastolic blood pressure of 104 placed her in acute danger.

It made sense on several levels for Patient E to measure her own blood pressure. Self-motivated self-monitoring not only generates more data points at different times of the day, but also avoids white coat hypertension and might avoid the costs of more frequent office visits.[11-13] She readily agreed. However, her health insurance did not pay for a home blood pressure monitor. The investigators used their own discretionary funds to pay the $90 needed to purchase one. That the costs of such machines are not covered by insurance reflects the limits of fee-for-service insurance as a method of paying for alternative approaches to good medical care.

Patient E was given a sheet on which to record her own blood pressure. She did more than was asked, taking her blood pressure several times a day. She became intrigued with the new knowledge generated by her home blood pressure measurements. She developed her own hypotheses about the causes of variation in her blood pressure. For instance, she thought the readings might be sensitive to stress at work. On March 17, the patient read her own blood pressure on her own manometer, and this was compared with the reading on the physician's office sphygmomanometer. Her reading was 145/102. The physician's reading was 148/102. Figure 5.3 displays the first two weeks of raw data as the patient collected them.

Figure 5.3 demonstrates several points. First, there is no easy way to build a mental model of a patient's blood pressure variation without statistical analysis. Even a simple run chart of the type displayed in Figures 5.1 and 5.2 yields more information than can be derived from the raw data as shown in Figure 5.3.

Second, a number of data points are missing. If this patient were admitted to a hospital for a study, one could ensure a complete set of

FIGURE 5.3 Raw Blood Pressure Data and Comments as Recorded by Patient E

Date	Time	7:00 AM	9:00 AM	11:00 AM	1:00 PM	3:00 PM	5:00 PM	7:00 PM	9:00 PM	11:00 PM	1:00 AM	Comments
2/15	Mon	130/97		144/93	142/99	149/97	142/92		— Sleep —		137/92	
2/16	Tues	132/95	132/94	127/88	149/93	117/84			— Sleep —		122/81	
2/17	Wed	129/82	142/99	139/98	150/88	135/93	144/94		— Sleep —		117/79 →L	did not take, last med. (V)
2/18	Thurs	139/95	133/91	128/87	139/92			153/113 (1st reading was 153/123)	— Sleep —		117/78 →R	company at 7:00, had not taken (C) yet
2/19	Fri	122/84	128/90		136/93	147/100				139/89		
2/20	Sat	119/84 →L 117/78 →R				107/76 →L 109/72 →R	133/90			126/82		did not take, last med (V)
2/21	Sun	118/84		142/98			126/80		— Sleep —		122/80	
2/22	Mon	124/87		143/101			149/89		— Sleep —		120/84	did not take, last med (V)

Date	Time	7:00 AM	9:00 AM	11:00 AM	1:00 PM	3:00 PM	5:00 PM	7:00 PM	9:00 PM	11:00 PM	1:00 AM	Comments
2/23	Tues	140/87	128/91		125/88		141/95		Sleep ——		118/80	
2/24	Wed	126/86		135/86			161/92		130/87			
2/25	Thurs	146/93		153/100		131/85		146/91				seminar and dinner after till 9:00
2/26	Fri	122/85		140/84		135/81						seminar and dinner after till 10:00
2/27	Sat		127/89			130/82					124/78	did not take last med (V)
2/28	Sun		120/84					128/81	120/79			did not take last med (V)
3/1	Mon	125/84			136/93	148/97		—— Sleep ——		104/68L	114/78	did not take last med (V)
3/2	Tues	130/91			118/84	125/84		154/102 — Company	102/72R	114/83	114/77 → ⌐	did not take last med (V)
											114/76 → ⌐	

Note: C = clonidine; V = verapamil

data with some effort. In the "real world," one must make do with what one has. Third, once developed, the model of Patient E's hypertension is for her alone. In comparison, literature will provide generalizations about populations, burying clinically meaningful individual variation in population averages (occasionally accompanied by standard deviations).

In Figure 5.3, note that the patient made comments that reflect her evolving mental model of her blood pressure. The comments are of two sorts: (1) explanations for missing her readings and (2) explanations for variance in the readings, such as not taking her medication. Good care is based on both the physician and the patient having an accurate and similar mental model of the condition. We think this is essential for good self-management and physician-patient partnership. To develop such a shared mental model, the next step is to create a run chart from these data points. The run chart for this patient over this time period is shown in Figure 5.4. This is a stable process in that only one data point is outside the control limits and no autocorrelation is obvious.[14] The patient's comments are recorded alongside the run chart. Sleeping beforehand seems to reduce blood pressure. Staying home and gardening seem to help. Working late, nights out at the bar, a social event, and lots of salt apparently do not help. We doubt that any internist would be surprised by this interpretation or think this was a great discovery, but that is not the point. Remember that this is a journey of discovery for the patient. Perhaps the discovery for the physician is that visiting the physician on March 17 (not shown) resulted in one of the highest recorded readings (white coat hypertension?).

This first run chart improved the partnership of the patient and her physician. Together, they learned:

1. Her blood pressure control was a stable process, with a median diastolic blood pressure of 88 mm Hg.

2. The patient grew more comfortable taking her blood pressure readings after the first three days, reflected in a lowering of her median diastolic blood pressure from an initial value of 93

FIGURE 5.4 Run Chart of Patient E's Diastolic Blood Pressure

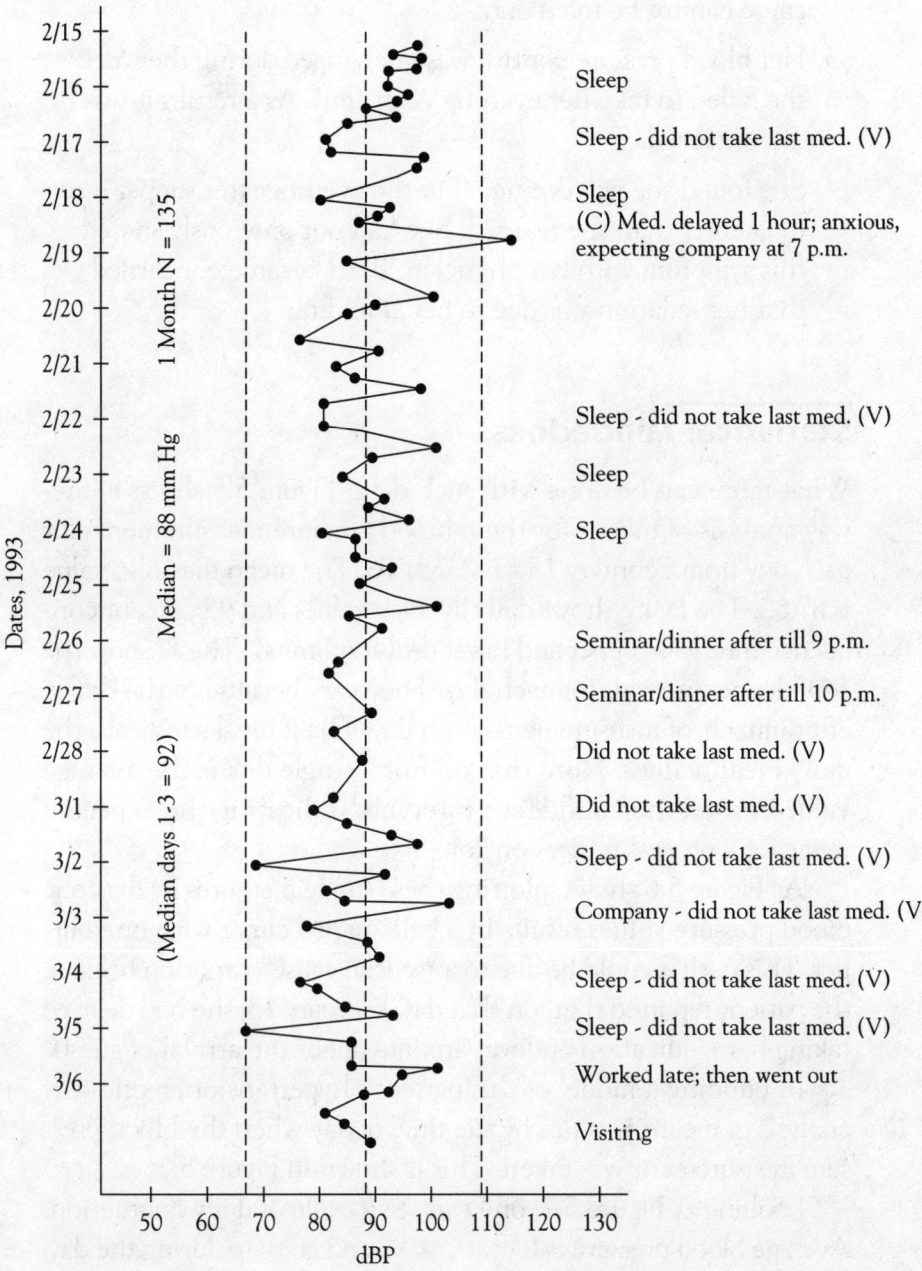

Note: C = clonidine; V = verapamil; "Sleep" refers to episodes when patient fell asleep involuntarily. Dashed lines are control limits.

mm Hg on the first three days. A change in technique as a cause cannot be ruled out.

3. Her blood pressure control was unchanged during the week she failed to take her evening verapamil. As a result, it was discontinued.

4. She found she was dozing off in the evening after supper more frequently than she realized. She had not previously shared this symptom with her physician. Both became concerned that her sedation was due to her clonidine.

Statistical Mindedness

What more can be done with such data? Figure 5.5 shows a one-way analysis of means for these blood pressure measurements for each day from February 15 to March 16. The mean diastolic value is 87.82. The figure shows daily average values and 95 percent confidence intervals (upper and lower decision limits). The I's show the confidence intervals for each day. They vary because of the different numbers of measurements each day. The asterisks indicate the daily mean values. Note that on not a single day is the average value beyond the confidence intervals, indicating the expected range for a process under control.

As Figure 5.6 shows, plotting these single measures by diastolic blood pressure values results in a bell-shaped curve with one outlier. This outlier could be due to a "special cause" variation because the patient reported that, on that day, February 18, she had delayed taking her medication and was anxious about the arrival of guests.

In building a model of this patient's hypertension, a one-way analysis of means was run by the time of day when the blood pressure measurement was taken. This is shown in Figure 5.7.

Looking at Figure 5.7, one can see a cycle of daily fluctuation. Average blood pressure is low at 7 A.M. and goes up during the day, reaching its highest average at 7 P.M., when it is at the upper 95 percent confidence limit. It is below these limits for 11 P.M. and 1 A.M. readings.

FIGURE 5.5 Mean Daily Diastolic Blood Pressure by Day, February 15 to March 16

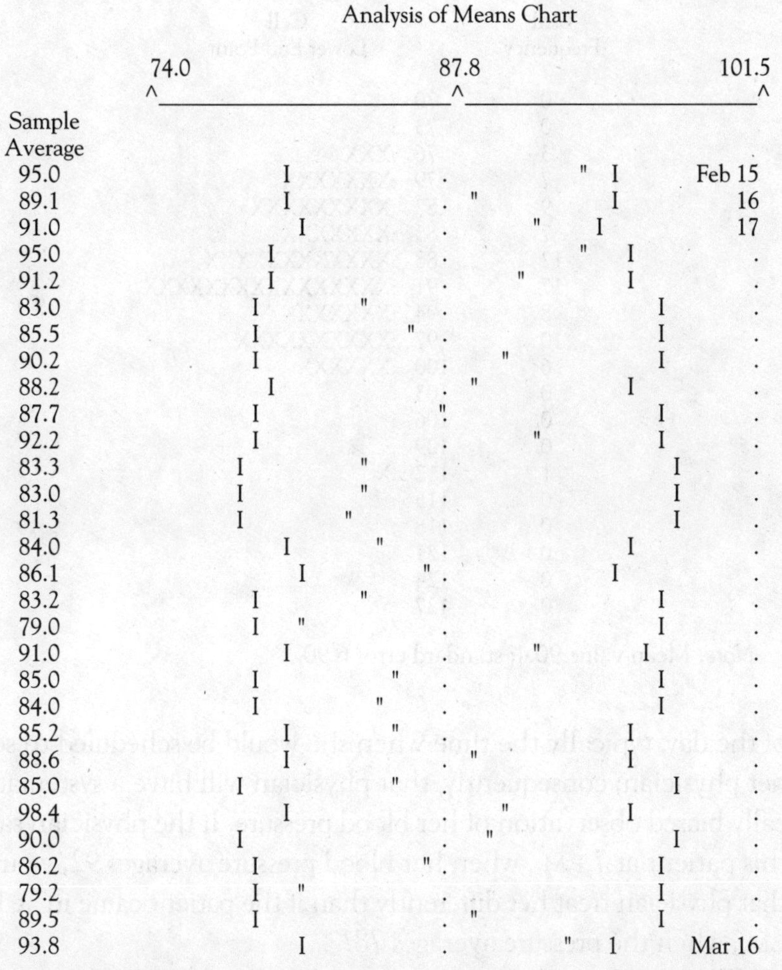

Analysis of Means Chart

```
            74.0                    87.8                      101.5
             ^                       ^                          ^
Sample
Average
95.0              I              .              "  I        Feb 15
89.1              I              .  "              I           16
91.0                I            .         "       I           17
95.0          I                  .              "  I           .
91.2          I                  .         "       I           .
83.0          I           "      .                    I        .
85.5          I              "   .                    I        .
90.2          I                  .      "             I        .
88.2             I               .   "             I           .
87.7          I               "  .                    I        .
92.2          I                  .      "             I        .
83.3       I           "         .                       I     .
83.0       I           "         .                       I     .
81.3       I        "            .                       I     .
84.0          I          "       .                    I        .
86.1           I              "  .                 I           .
83.2       I           "         .                    I        .
79.0       I     "               .                    I        .
91.0          I                  .         "       I           .
85.0       I              "      .                    I        .
84.0       I              "      .                    I        .
85.2       I              "      .                 I           .
88.6       I                     .     "           I           .
85.0       I                  "  .                 I           .
98.4          I                  .         "       I           .
90.0       I                     .   "                I        .
86.2       I                  "  .                 I           .
79.2       I  "                  .                 I           .
89.5       I                     .  "              I           .
93.8          I                  .              "  1        Mar 16
```

Note: Overall mean diastolic blood pressure 87.8. Upper and lower 95 percent confidence intervals shown for each day (I).

That blood pressure varies systematically throughout the day probably has been known since the time when Harvey Cushing first brought blood pressure measurement to the United States in the 1900s. Daily variation, however, is not the point. We are building a mental model for this patient, helping her understand her own condition. Her blood pressure is higher than average in the middle

FIGURE 5.6 Frequency Plot Diastolic Blood Pressure Measures for
Patient E

Cell Frequency	Cell Lower End Point	
0	70	:
0	73	:
3	76	:XXX
7	79	:XXXXXXX
9	82	:XXXXXXXXX
7	85	:XXXXXXX
12	88	:XXXXXXXXXXXX
17	91	:XXXXXXXXXXXXXXXXX
8	94	:XXXXXXXX
10	97	:XXXXXXXXXX
6	100	:XXXXXX
0	103	:
0	106	:
0	109	:
1	112	:X
0	115	:
0	118	:
0	121	:
0	124	:
0	127	:

Note: Mean value 90.4; standard error 6.90.

of the day, typically the time when she would be scheduled to see
her physician; consequently, that physician will have a systematically biased observation of her blood pressure. If the physician saw
this patient at 7 P.M., when her blood pressure averages 92, would
that physician treat her differently than if the patient came in at 11
P.M., when the pressure averages 78?

Without the patient as a partner, the physician could—and in
this case did—misjudge the patient's condition.

What about the effect of medication for this patient? In February, the patient stopped her evening verapamil, and no difference
in blood pressure resulted. In April, she stopped her evening clonidine from time to time, but this change did affect her blood pressure the next day. This is shown in Figure 5.8. This figure is
important because it shows how this patient carried out her own

FIGURE 5.7 Mean Diastolic Blood Pressure by Hour of the Day for Patient E

```
                78.0                        87.7                       97.3
                 ^                            ^                          ^
Sub-    Value    _____|_____
group   UDL
LDL
 86                            I      "                 I   7AM
 84      91

 98               I                          "                  I   9AM
 81      93

 92               I                          "          I   11AM
 82      93

 89                    I                "               I   1PM
 83      92

 88                    I            "               I   3PM
 83      91

 91                   I                     "          I   5PM
 82      92

 92                   I                     "      7PM
 83      92

 89                   I                    "      9PM
 75     100

 78            I                                  I   11PM
 81      94

 82                "                                I   1AM
 83      91
```

Note: One-way analysis of means 95 percent; upper and lower confidence intervals (I); overall mean value 87.7; hour of day shown on the right; mean values for each hour and values for lower and upper limits shown on the left.

quantitative, controlled clinical trial. Without medication, the next day's mean value was 92.7; with medication, it was 86.4. "I don't need all this statistical analysis to tell me this," the skeptical physician might say.

FIGURE 5.8 Next Day Readings with and Without Clonidine, Showing the Effect of This Medication on Diastolic Blood Pressure

Analysis of Means Chart

	80.7	90.7	100.7
	^	^	^
Sample			
Average			
92.7		l . "	No pm CL
86.4	" I	. I	Took pm CL

Here is what we consider to be the value of such careful quantitative analysis:

1. Patients learn for themselves about their particular condition and how to control it.
2. The physician and the patient learn that the effect of this medication is a six-point difference in blood pressure.
3. The physician and the patient can avoid the temptation to tamper with a process that is under control when they observe a special cause disturbance, such as white coat hypertension.
4. The effect of one regimen can be compared with others, such as exercise, reducing stress, or using other medications.

We think a patient should be able to ask and get an answer to this question: "I get these side effects from this medication, which I don't like. Is it worth this discomfort to get a six-point reduction in my blood pressure?" Perhaps a good answer might sound like this: "If you can sleep or rest from 5:30 to 6:30 P.M., you can bring your average blood pressure down by four points. Therefore, your net loss is an average of two points. A two-point difference will result in an average life expectancy increase of four months for people like you, but it also will reduce the chance that you will need bypass surgery. However, if you both rest and take your medication, you can get a ten-point reduction, and that will really make a difference. It's up to you."

A good mental model shared by patient and physician must be quantitative. It allows for better-reasoned trade-offs, such as those provided more formally by decision analysis.

By grouping the values week by week, one can get a better understanding of how this patient is progressing. Eighteen weeks of average blood pressure measurements are shown in Figure 5.9. By the third week, this patient was able to bring her blood pressure down from 90 to 85. During the sixth to twelfth weeks, the patient experimented with reducing her medication intake to see whether she could avoid side effects. By the last six weeks, she had found a way to keep her blood pressure below her previous average.

Now turn to the one-way analysis of means for the standard deviations in her blood pressure (Figure 5.10). One of the foundations of CQI is to reduce variation.

Notice that the weekly samples have standard deviations ranging from a high of 8.3 to a low of 3.0. Her third week, with a low average blood pressure, was achieved with a high standard deviation. Her later lower means were achieved with smaller standard deviations. Low means and low variation around those means achieve the CQI definition of an improved process that is under control; that is, her blood pressure is more stable and lower.

Discussion

The patient (P. L.) wrote the following about her perception of this new participatory care:

> I am a forty-eight-year-old female and have been diagnosed with hypertension since I was approximately thirty-five. My mother has hypertension, and I was just recently informed that my father's brothers and sisters, of which there are six, all suffer from either hypertension or heart problems.
>
> I have seen several doctors over this period of time and have always felt that the treatment I have received in the form of prescribed medications has not been adequate. On

FIGURE 5.9 One-Way Analysis of Means for Patient E, Mean Values by Week for Eighteen Weeks

Analysis of Means Chart

```
            79.2                       89.6                      99.9
             ^                          ^                         ^
Sample
Average
 90.6                             I      .    "    I
 87.1                           I    "   .         I
 85.0                         "  I       .         I
 87.9                           I    "   .         I
 88.1                           I    "   .         I
 93.4                           I         .             "
 90.9                         I          .    "    I
 89.9                         I          .    "    I
 93.0                       I             .      "   I
 96.9                       I            .         I       "
 95.7                     I              .         I   "
 93.0              I                      .      "            I
 88.1                           I    "   .         I
 87.4                         I   "      .         I
 87.9                         I    "     .             I
 87.9                       I        "   .             I
 90.4                     I              .    "               I
 85.4                     I               .                   I
```

Note: Overall mean blood pressure 89.62; overall standard deviation 6.206; upper and lower 95 percent confidence intervals shown (I).

the infrequent occasions that I was able to have my blood pressure taken, it was always higher than would be expected, given my medication. I did realize, however, that just knowing I would have my pressure read was stressful, as I anticipated a high reading.

This constant concern is a part of my nature, and try as I might, I cannot seem to "NOT WORRY ABOUT IT," as everyone advises me. It wasn't until I started this program and became very accustomed to taking my own pressure that I felt I had any control at all. I knew that all my prescribed medication has been based on what I can only refer to as "hyper readings," but I never had any control over it.

FIGURE 5.10 One-Way Analysis of Standard Deviations for Patient E

Analysis of Standard Deviations Chart

```
        0               6.2                                    28.6
        ^_____^_____^
Sample
Average
  7.5        I        .     "  I
  5.8        I     " .          I
  8.3        I        .      "  I
  6.5        I        "       I
  7.9        I        .      "  I
  5.3        I     "  .         I
  5.6        I     " .          I
  4.9        I     "  .         I
  4.7        I   "    .         I
  5.9        I      "           I
------
  3.0     "  I           .      I
  4.7        I   "       .      I
  4.0        I  "        .      I
  4.9        I      "    .      I
  4.6        I    "      .      I
  4.4        I    "      .      I
  5.3        I    "      .      I
```

Note: Overall mean blood pressure 89.62; overall standard deviation 6.206; upper and lower 95 percent confidence intervals shown (I).

Over the past months, I have been taking my pressure whenever I could and have been recording it on a graph. I can see patterns and the results of my lifestyle reflected on these records. As a result, I am much more in control, and I am able to determine what affects my readings. I also feel that my medication is much more accurate, given the fact that Dr. Headrick has this information and not just my "hyper readings." All of this, of course, is a great source of comfort to me, and, again, helps me to keep my pressure down. I'm quite certain that I would be on a much higher dosage if it were not for this program.

This also brings up the matter of changing medications. We are now in a much better position to determine the effects of new medications, and I am very willing to try new ones, where I never was before. Any trial on a different medication was always stressful for me. I am much better now because I can see right away how it's working for me.

What I have to work on now is taking the initiative to make improvements in my lifestyle. I can see how exercise and diet affect me. I need to become motivated to make changes and lose weight. Right now, I am disappointed with myself for not moving forward in that direction, and I know this concern will show up on my chart.

I am grateful that I've had this opportunity and feel that I'm so much more in touch with my problem. I sincerely hope that I can live up to my end of the deal.

It is our belief that CQI leads to a very different way of thinking about good care. A patient with an accurate mental model, who carries out experiments to know how treatment affects her condition and who can consider the trade-offs against her personal goals, should define the standard of good care. Patients who have achieved this state can self-manage their care and reduce the costs of professional care, perhaps by reducing the frequency of office visits. Patient E's visits have been reduced from every four weeks to every twelve weeks.

Patient E was recruited, in part, because her blood pressure was difficult to control, even on three medications. The approach described here had several effects, some immediate.

1. She was no longer afraid to have her blood pressure taken. In fact, controlling the process herself is reflected by lower blood pressure after the first week.

2. Evidence of her high blood pressure at the time of her visits allowed the physician to recognize the role of white coat hypertension and to begin reducing medications. Previously, medications were being added, with higher costs and greater side effects.

3. Her mean diastolic blood pressure on her current two-medicine regimen is 91 mm Hg. The physician and the patient agree that this is acceptable, given the side effects of increased medication dosage. This capacity of the patient-physician team to make quantitative trade-offs in care choices should be a measure of good care.

4. She recognizes the effect of stress and exercise, so she does not overreact when a change in blood pressure results from these causes. She previously "panicked" when her blood pressure went up. Likewise, she sees the difference in her blood pressure when she exercises regularly, reinforcing the need to continue.

5. Because of this effort, the monthly cost of her medication is estimated to have dropped from $62.50 a month to $30.99 per month. (The exact costs for this patient are unavailable. Prices quoted were obtained from a local discount pharmacy.)

6. This patient now has a mental model of her condition that includes nine variables: measurement error, variation from day to day, time of day, anxiety, sleep and relaxation, salt intake, clonidine, verapamil, and white coat hypertension. She also says she is willing to continue to try new approaches, thus adding to her model. This model is shared with her physician.

It is possible that patients will be more able and willing to adapt to this new partnership than physicians. A variation will occur in patients' willingness to participate. On the basis of our experience with these five patients, we offer the following predictors. Participation is more likely if:

1. High blood pressure is a major concern. The patient is willing to spend the time monitoring his or her own blood pressure.

2. Patients have labile blood pressure that changes rapidly with

external factors. (The literature suggests that approximately 20 percent of patients with mid-to-moderate hypertension have white coat hypertension.[9,10])

3. Patients have blood pressure that is not easily controlled with minimal side effects by the usual methods.

In the future, good care for hypertension will not be measured by the prestige of the hospital or the years of training of the physician. We believe that excellent care for hypertension can be measured as follows. An outsider asks this question of a representative patient (or patients): "When you take your 5 P.M. blood pressure readings, other things being equal, what percentage reduction do you get in your diastolic blood pressure after exercise?" The ability of the patient to give an accurate quantitative answer to this question defines a standard of excellent care we might aspire to.

In this chapter, we have posed a series of questions that are worth raising and answering:

How do we know this approach will be better? So far, we have shown what is possible and some evidence as to the circumstances in which this approach will work. It seems to us that a more formal trial is the next step. *Can a patient build a good mental model without statistical analysis?* We don't think so.

We included a statistician expert in quality control (W.K.) as part of our team. *Does a physician need a quality consultant for every patient?* That would be impossible. We need to simplify the methods so that any patient and physician can use them. Developing software that a ten-year-old could use is a good aspiration.

Would run charts alone do perfectly well for the average patient? The reader should look at the data as they unfold in this chapter. *How many data and how much analysis are needed to understand this patient's blood pressure?*

Is less variability associated with better outcomes? With respect to blood pressure, is the greater variation in Figure 5.2 better or worse than in Figure 5.1? We don't know.

A suggested research agenda might include the following:

1. Continue the partnership with this and other patients.

2. Find out how many patients are willing and able to become partners in this way.

3. Develop easy-to-use software for patient and physician.

4. Change medical education on a pilot basis to increase physicians' ability to collect and analyze data such as these.

5. Carry out a formal trial of usual care for hypertension versus partnership care, measuring blood pressure control, patient knowledge, and costs as outcomes.

Notes

1. Mellins, R. B., Evans, D., Zimmerman, B., & Clark, N. M. (1992). Patient compliances: Are we wasting our time and don't know it? *American Review of Respiratory Disease, 146*, 1376–1377.

2. Headrick, L., Neuhauser, D., Melnikow, J., et al. (1991). Introducing continuous quality improvement thinking to medical students. *Quality Review Bulletin, 17*(8), 254–260.

3. Headrick, L., Neuhauser, D., & Melnikow, J. (1992). Teaching medical students about quality and costs of care at Case Western Reserve University. *Academic Medicine, 67*(3), 157–159.

4. Neuhauser, D., Headrick, L., & Miller, D. (1992). The best asthma care: A case problem in continuous quality improvement. *Quality Assurance and Utilization Review, 7*(3), 76–80.

5. Headrick, L., Neuhauser, D., & Melnikow, J. (1993). Asthma health status: Ongoing measurement in the context of continuous quality improvement. *Medical Care, 31*(Suppl. 3), MS97–MS105.

6. Headrick, L., Neuhauser, D., Melnikow, J., Vanek, E., Miller, D., & Christie, R. (1993). Quality and cost of asthma care: The CWRU Cleveland Asthma Project. In N. Goldfield, M. Pine, & J. Pine (Eds.), *Measuring and managing health care quality* (pp. 5:15–5:23). Gaithersburg, MD: Aspen Publishers.

7. Greenfield, S., Kaplan, S. H., Ware, J. E., Yano, E. M., & Frank, H.J.L. (1988). Patient's participation in medical care: Effects on

blood sugar control and quality of life in diabetes. *Journal of General Internal Medicine, 3,* 448–457.

8. Weber, M. A., & Drayer, J. M. (1978). Role of blood pressure monitoring in the diagnosis of hypertension. *Journal of Hypertension,* 4(Suppl. 5), 5325–5327.

9. Stahl, S. M., Kelley, C. R., Neill, P. J., Grimm, C. E., & Mamlin, J. (1984). Effects of home blood pressure measurement on long-term BP control. *American Journal of Public Health, 74,* 704–709.

10. Mejia, A. D., Egan, B. M., Schorle, N. J., & Zweifler, A. J. (1990). Artifacts in measurement of blood pressure and lack of target organ involvement in the assessment of patients with treatment-resistant hypertension. *Annals of Internal Medicine, 112,* 270–277.

11. Soghlician, K., Casper, S. M., Firement, B. H., Hunkeler, E. M., et al. (1992). Home blood pressure monitoring: Effect on use of medical services and medical care costs. *Medical Care, 30,* 855–865.

12. Mejia, A. D., Julius, S., Jones, K. A., Schorle, N. T., & Kneisley, J. (1990). The Tecumseh Blood Pressure Study: Normative data in blood pressure self-determination. *Archives of Internal Medicine, 150,* 1209–1213.

13. Pickering, T. G., James, G. D., Boddie, C., Harshfield, G. A., et al. (1988). How common is white coat hypertension? *Journal of the American Medical Association, 114,* 975–928.

14. Hamada, M., Mackay, R. J., & Whitney, J. B. (1993). Continuous process improvement with observational studies. *Journal of Quality Technology, 25*(2), 77–84.

6

Blood Pressure Variability

Beyond the State of the Art

Glenn L. Laffel, M.D., Ph.D.

This chapter rests upon two underlying premises. First, much is known about blood pressure variability in clinically stable, ambulatory patients. Second, inexpensive medical technologies and statistical methods are available that would enable physicians to extend their knowledge about blood pressure variability to an entirely new frontier: the acute care setting. These same technologies and statistical methods could almost certainly be applied to dozens of other physiological variables that are routinely monitored in acute care settings. Examples are heart rate, temperature, respiratory rate, oxygen saturation, central venous pressure, and urine output. Arterial blood pressure, however, serves as a useful case to illustrate the potential and utility of the particular tools that are the subject of this discussion.

Physicians and patients prefer to think about blood pressure as a constant variable. This straightforward approach is encouraged by epidemiological and insurance data that demonstrate a correlation between blood pressure readings obtained in physicians' offices and the risk of developing systemic complications from hypertension.

Despite these views, members of the medical community have known for more than 250 years that blood pressure actually varies from beat to beat. Steven Hales first demonstrated this fact in horses in the early 1700s.[1] The modern era for the study of blood pressure variability began in 1969 when Sir George Pickering and colleagues developed a technique to monitor ambulatory intra-arterial blood pressure in humans.[2] This technique and the more recent advent of twenty-four-hour noninvasive monitoring devices have enabled researchers to identify cyclical trends in blood pressure that are associated with sleep and wakefulness, and more rapid, situational changes associated with various environmental stimuli.[3-5]

Investigators have explored many aspects of blood pressure variability in ambulatory, clinically stable patients.[6-10] This well-developed line of research has confirmed the variability in blood pressure and has sharpened the debate surrounding the diagnosis and prognosis of hypertension. The objectives of this chapter are to review briefly what is known about blood pressure variability in ambulatory, clinically stable patients and to propose that, with the benefit of some newly available technologies and statistical methods, this knowledge could be extended to new areas, such as the acute care setting. For a more detailed review of the subject of blood pressure variability, the reader is referred to the review article by Floras.[11]

Readers familiar with the managerial paradigm of quality management will easily recognize the strong parallels between the biomedical approach to variability described in this chapter and the manufacturing-based approach to variability developed by Deming, Juran, and others. A full discussion of such similarities is beyond the scope of this chapter. However, it appears that two aspects of the approaches developed in industrial settings actually could enhance the traditional biomedical approach to variability. First, industrial techniques include statistical tools to analyze serial data from production processes. These tools, falling under the general heading of "statistical process control" (SPC), may prove useful in analyzing serial patient-related data. Second, industrial approaches to variability encourage broad thinking about causes of variability in complex systems. When applied to the subject of blood pressure variability, for example, the industrial model encourages joint consideration of environmental factors, physicians' decisions, educational processes for physicians and patients, patient preferences, the availability and cost of blood pressure treatments, and other factors, in addition to considering the physiological issues that are the standard focus of the biomedical model. The breadth and analytical power of industrial methods to understand variability in complex systems are prodigious. Although in this chapter I concentrate on their applicability to increase understanding of physiological processes, additional uses of the industrial model should be kept in mind.

Defining Blood Pressure Variability

Physicians routinely observe variability in serial recordings of their patients' blood pressure. Thus, their ability to provide optimal care depends on their ability to interpret this variability. For example, the correct interpretation of blood pressure differences across a series of clinic visits[12] is critical to the diagnosis of hypertension and the assessment of responsiveness to therapy. As another example, an awareness of the effects of posture and exercise on blood pressure is required to identify those who are being treated too aggressively or too conservatively.

In all likelihood, members of the medical community need to agree on the definition of blood pressure variability and the appropriate methodologies by which to quantify it before one can assess whether physicians respond appropriately when they encounter such variability. Unfortunately, the striking recent trend has been to create ever more definitions and quantification methods that apply to blood pressure variability. Among definitions proposed are[11]: differences between mean clinic and ambulatory blood pressure[6,7]; peak-trough differences (the range of blood pressure recordings over a one-day period); differences between mean waking and sleeping blood pressures; differences between mean blood pressures recorded at thirty-minute intervals; the variance or standard deviation of all, or a sample of all readings over one day[3,5,10,13-15]; the coefficient of variation of variability data; the root of the mean squared successive differences[16]; and more recently, results of spectral analysis of blood pressure variability.[17]

The presence of two conflicting needs has prevented those in the medical community from reaching consensus about the most appropriate definition of blood pressure variability. On the one hand, clinicians—who already are besieged by clinical information—need concise, easily interpretable and applicable information on variability. On the other hand, clinicians need valid and reliable information, and this need, in turn, requires the use of rather complex, analytical methods that can account for autocorrelation in observations, cycles, trends, or other phenomena associated with complex biological systems. These more complex methods produce data that are less easily interpretable than those produced by more simplistic but less accurate approaches to understanding variability.

The approach used by Floras's group, among others[11,18], appears to strike a reasonable balance: they use frequency distributions to display blood pressure recordings that they have recorded from a patient over a twenty-four-hour period (Figure 6.1). In addition, they derive the mean blood pressure from all beats that occur while subjects are awake, derive the standard deviation about this value, and then use this standard deviation as an index of blood pressure variability.[3,13,15,19] Using this approach with healthy individuals, Floras's group found that variability tends to be 10 to 15 percent of the mean blood pressure. (This approach may not be optimal in acute care settings, however. In such settings, discussed below, real-time assessment of blood pressure trends and blood pressure variability are required in order to have an impact on patient care.)

Diurnal Variations in Blood Pressure

A systemic, easily detectable component of blood pressure variability is diurnal variability (Figure 6.2), in which mean blood pressure during sleep decreases by 20 to 25 percent, as compared with average waking blood pressure. Studies have shown that sleep itself, not the time at which sleep occurs, is associated with these blood

FIGURE 6.1 Frequency Distribution of Diastolic (left) and Systolic (right) Blood Pressures During One Twenty-Four-Hour Period of Intra-Arterial Blood Pressure Monitoring in a Single Subject

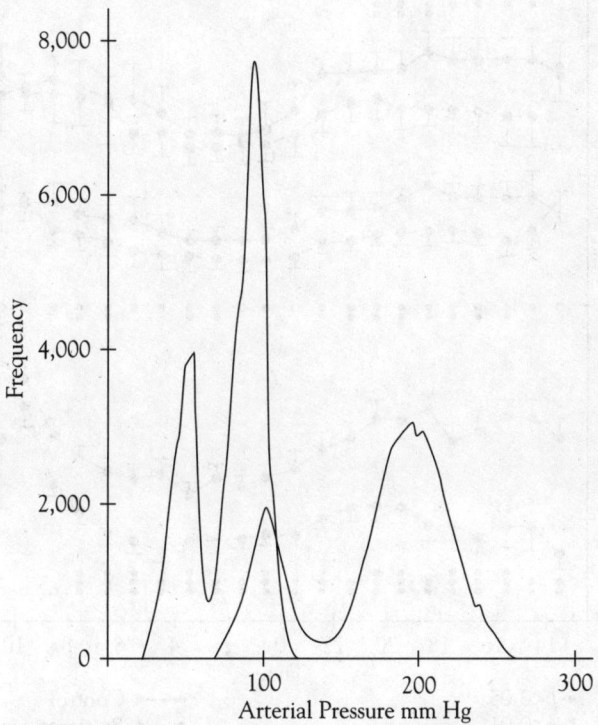

Note: The frequency distribution is bimodal for both systolic and diastolic pressures because the effect of sleep produces a lower mode in each case.

Source: Littler, W. A., & Komsuoglu, B. (1989). Which is the most accurate method of measuring blood pressure? *American Heart Journal, 117,* p. 725. Reprinted by permission.

pressure reductions. Thus, people who work at night exhibit reductions in blood pressure during their daytime sleep.

Physiological Control of Blood Pressure

The neurohumoral, vascular, and respiratory systems all play key roles in affecting mean blood pressure and its beat-to-beat variability,[5,20] but it is the neurohumoral system that mediates the afore-

FIGURE 6.2 Hourly Trend Plots of Mean (± SD) Hourly Systolic and Diastolic Blood Pressures and Heart Rate Recording

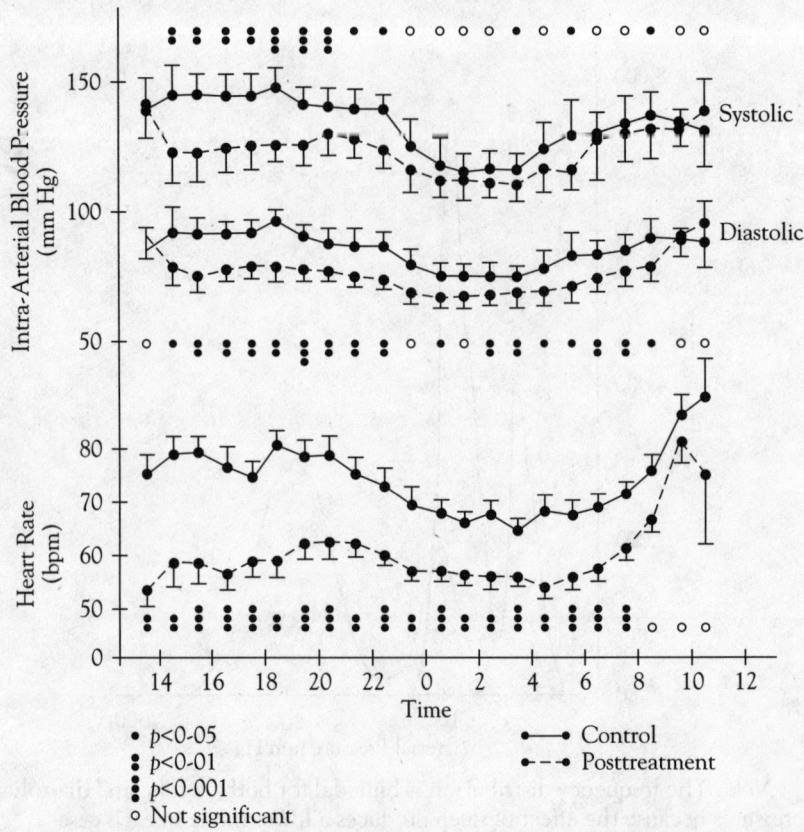

Note: Recordings were made in eight patients before and three months after long-term treatment with the beta-blocking drug metoprolol. The diurnal pattern of blood pressure is maintained during treatment, with the most significant reduction of blood pressure during the waking period.

Source: From Littler, W. A., & Komsuoglu, B. (1989). Which is the most accurate method of measuring blood pressure? *American Heart Journal, 117,* p. 726. Reprinted by permission.

mentioned diurnal variations in blood pressure.[12,21] Increased outflow from the sympathetic nervous system precedes the rise in blood pressure that begins shortly before sleep ends.[5] Sympathetic antagonists block this rise. The parasympathetic nervous system probably also contributes to neurohumoral control:

most investigators have shown that the parasympatholytic agent atropine decreases blood pressure and blood pressure variability.[22] Neurohumoral systems also mediate blood pressure elevations associated with exercise and emotion, in addition to their key role in mediating diurnal blood pressure variation, and they probably underlie the "white coat hypertension phenomenon" discussed below.

Both the sympathetic and parasympathetic nervous systems are triggered by baroreceptor reflexes centered in the brain. In addition, the increased blood pressure variability associated with increasing age and high mean blood pressure is almost certainly related to defective baroreflex control.[19]

Loss of normal vascular compliance, as is commonly seen with advancing age, also contributes to increased blood pressure variability. "Stiff" arteries are unable to dampen the effects of beat-to-beat variability in cardiac output, and this inability translates into increased beat-to-beat variability in blood pressure. Respiratory contributions to blood pressure variability are short-lived and are mediated through the parasympathetic nervous system and through changing venous return to the heart.

Noninvasive Measurement of Blood Pressure

Sphygmomanometers

Sphygmomanometers—time-honored tools—are by far the most commonly used to measure blood pressure. The use of a sphygmomanometer to obtain blood pressure readings has become one of the most widely accepted traditions of modern clinical medicine. Sphygmomanometers are easy to use and provide information of obvious clinical value.

However, sphygmomanometers cannot measure blood pressure as precisely as direct intra-arterial recordings; even when they are used by skilled practitioners under ideal conditions, auscultatory readings do not capture beat-to-beat variation in blood pressure and tend to underestimate systolic blood pressure and to overestimate diastolic blood pressure, both by an average of eight mm Hg.[23] Furthermore, sphygmomanometry is rarely used under ideal conditions in general practice. Real-life factors that further confound blood pressure measurement by sphygmomanometers include the use of different observers or different sphygmomanometers in serial office visits, the making of serial recordings at different times of the day, and the failure to standardize the patient's position (reclining, sitting, or standing) or the length of rest preceding the recording.

One cause of measurement error is particularly difficult to eliminate: the anxiety response engendered by the recorder, particularly if he or she is a physician. For example, Mancia and others[24] reported systolic/diastolic elevations associated with so-called white coat hypertension to be as high as 27/15 mm Hg above baseline. Of note, Mancia's group found that the last of four measurements over a ten-minute period much more closely approximated the patient's true baseline.

Most physicians are aware of the risk of measurement error associated with standard sphygmomanometry, so they tend to make recordings on two or three separate visits before making definitive decisions regarding treatment. Some investigators suggest that blood pressure recordings be obtained on six separate visits before deciding whether a patient has elevated blood pressure.[18] Another approach to overcome this risk of measurement error is to train patients to record their own blood pressure at home. Studies of home blood pressure recordings have shown that they average six to ten mm Hg lower than those obtained by physicians.[25]

Ambulatory Blood Pressure Monitors

Ambulatory blood pressure monitors are portable, relatively inexpensive devices that can be affixed to a subject's arm and used to record blood pressure automatically at preset intervals. They have spread throughout medical practice during the past decade. As a result, clinicians can now easily obtain information regarding their patients' blood pressure during normal daily activities. These monitors are ideal tools to rule out white coat hypertension because blood pressure is recorded automatically, far from the doctor's office.

Ambulatory blood pressure monitors, however, use the same noninvasive technology as sphygmomanometers, so they potentially are subject to several of the same limitations. White and his group[26] compared blood pressure observations obtained from ambulatory blood pressure recorders with simultaneous recordings from intra-arterial catheters and pressure transducers. They found a strong correlation between the results obtained by the invasive and noninvasive methods. The researchers concluded that most of the ambulatory blood pressure monitors provide reliable information in patients who are resting but that some types of monitors are better than others at recording blood pressure during strenuous activity.

Documenting this strong correlation is an important contribution, but the above study does not address whether ambulatory blood pressure monitors can be used to accurately quantify blood pressure variability. The question is important because blood pressure is essentially a continuous variable, whereas most ambulatory monitors measure blood pressure approximately once every fifteen minutes. How frequently must blood pressure be measured, and how big must the sample size be to accurately assess blood pressure variability with accuracy?

To address this question, Di Rienzo and his group calculated the average systolic, diastolic, and mean blood pressure from continuous intra-arterial recordings in twenty ambulatory hypertensive patients and compared these values with those calculated by averaging the results of isolated blood pressure recordings spaced five, ten, fifteen, thirty, or sixty minutes apart.[14] In each subject, the mean values calculated from the continuous data collection closely corresponded to the mean values calculated by the intermittent method. However, the blood pressure variability determined by the intermittent analysis differed significantly from that calculated by using the continuous record, especially when sampling frequencies were greater than every fifteen minutes. This analysis needs to be confirmed in larger populations of ambulatory patients. In the meantime, it is likely that ambulatory blood pressure monitors that infrequently sample blood pressure will not be regarded as optimal tools for the assessment of blood pressure variability.

Clinical Significance of Variability in Blood Pressure

Information regarding blood pressure variability may be useful in diagnosing hypertension,[6,8,27] assessing its prognosis,[9] and measuring the effects of antihypertensive drugs.[13,28,29]

Diagnosing Hypertension

Most clinicians diagnose hypertension in patients who have blood pressure values greater than 140/90 mm Hg.[27] However, they also recognize that blood pressure is inherently variable and that this diagnosis carries a lifelong commitment to reduce blood pressure (with its associated costs and potential side effects). Therefore, clinicians tend to be conservative in establishing the diagnosis.

Several investigators have presented evidence that supports this conservative approach. For example, Mancia's group[30] sorted 175 patients into normotensive, borderline hypertensive, moderate hypertensive, and severe hypertensive groups by using World Health Organization (WHO) criteria for clinic diastolic blood pressure and found that the twenty-four-hour mean blood pressure measured intra-arterially exhibited significant scatter and overlap between groups (Figure 6.3). As another example, many investigators have reported that the blood pressure of more than 25 percent of patients who are apparently hypertensive at baseline becomes completely normal when the patient takes placebo therapy.[31] A likely explanation for this phenomenon is that many subjects enter clinical trials after having been incorrectly diagnosed in the first place. These studies suggest that an optimal approach to the diagnosis of hypertension should include a careful assessment of blood pressure variability and that isolated blood pressure recordings (even two or three) do not provide sufficient grounds for the diagnosis.

FIGURE 6.3 The Twenty-Four-Hour Mean Arterial Pressure Values in 175 Subjects Who Underwent Intra-Arterial Monitoring

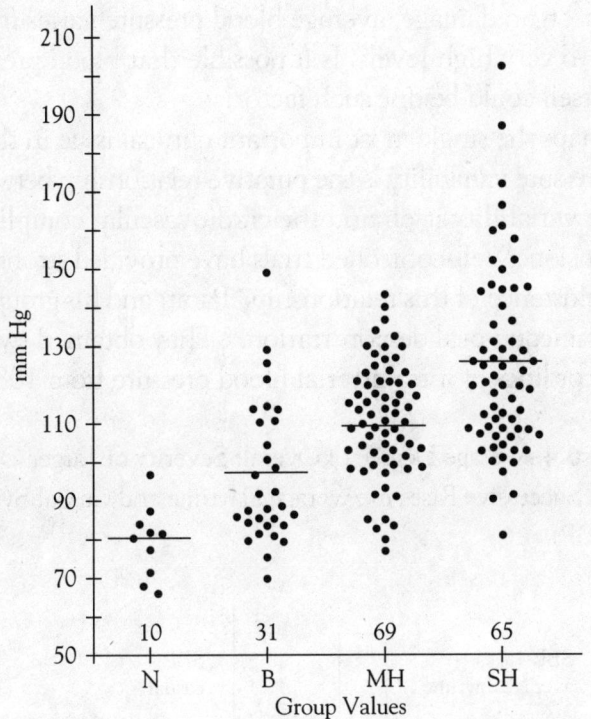

Note: Clinic diastolic blood pressure < 90 mm Hg = normotensive (N); > 90 and < 95 mm Hg = borderline hypertensive (B); > 95 and < 110 mm Hg = moderately hypertensive (MH); > 110 mm Hg = severely hypertensive (SH). The bars show the average twenty-four-hour values for each group.

Source: From Mancia, G., Parati, G., Albini, F., & Villani, A. (1988). Circadian blood pressure variations and their impact on disease. *Journal of Cardiovascular Pharmacology, 12*(Suppl. 7), S11–S17. Reprinted by permission.

Assessing Prognosis of Hypertension

Studies using ambulatory blood pressure monitoring devices have shown that the average twenty-four-hour blood pressure is more closely related to the cardiovascular sequelae of hypertension than are isolated clinic blood pressure readings[9,32–34] (Figure 6.4). This finding supports the notion, discussed previously, that casually obtained blood pressure readings do not precisely reflect ambient blood pressure in many patients. However, these studies also revealed that other factors must be playing a role: within each class of target organ damage, average blood pressure varies from nearly normal to very high levels. Is it possible that blood pressure variability itself could be one such factor?

Perhaps the single most important clinical issue in the study of blood pressure variability is the putative relationship between blood pressure variability itself and the cardiovascular complications of hypertension. Well-controlled trials have provided strong evidence for the existence of this relationship.[8] Parati and his group provided the first unequivocal demonstration.[10] They obtained twenty-four-hour recordings of intra-arterial blood pressure from 108 hospital-

FIGURE 6.4 Average Degree of Overall Severity of Target Organ Damage with Successive Rises in Average Daytime and Casual Systolic Pressures (SBP)

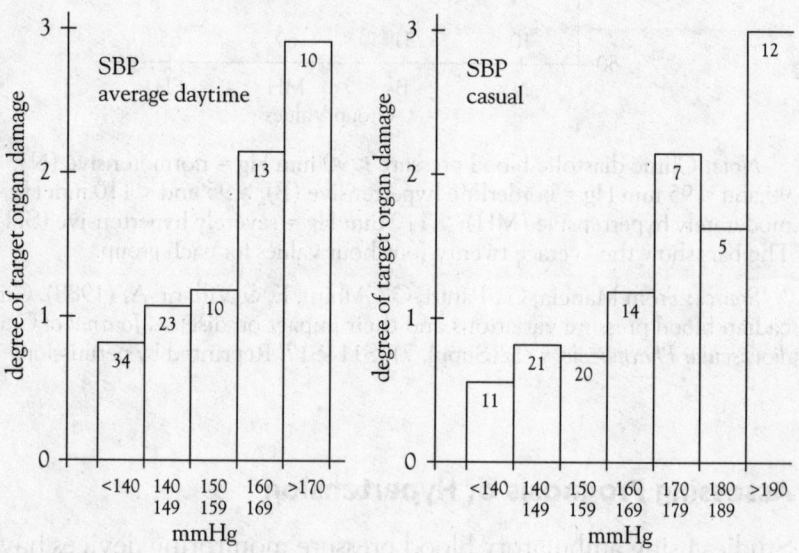

Source: From Pessina, A. C., Palatini, P., Sperti, G., and others. (1985). Evaluation of hypertension and related target organ damage by average daytime blood pressure. *Clinical Experiments in Hypertension, [A]7*, p. 271. Reprinted by courtesy of Marcel Dekker, Inc.

ized patients with essential hypertension and sorted patients into five groups based on their mean twenty-four-hour blood pressure. Within each group, they created two subgroups according to the magnitude of the blood pressure variability (expressed as the standard deviation of the twenty-four-hour blood pressure mean). Then, using fundoscopic examinations, chest radiography, and reviews of electrocardiograms to assess the long-term sequelae of increased blood pressure, Parati and colleagues found that, in all five groups, the subgroup with lower blood pressure variability had a lower prevalence and severity of target organ damage (Figure 6.5). Palatini and his group[35] conducted a study using noninvasive techniques; they recently published a preliminary report that documents a similar correlation in a larger series of patients ($n = 522$). Other investigators have provided indirect support for this finding as well.[36-38]

To further investigate a possible causal relationship between blood pressure variability and the cardiovascular sequelae of hypertension, one would need to develop a well-tolerated drug that specifically blunts blood pressure variability. Unfortunately, studies have shown that currently available antihypertensive medications do not have this specific effect.[39-41]

Measuring the Effects of Antihypertensive Drugs

When assessing the effects of antihypertensive medications, the challenge is to detect sustained, significant hypotensive effects that are superimposed upon normal levels of blood pressure variability. Ambulatory blood pressure monitors are ideal for such assessments because they provide reproducible, consistent results and a relatively rich set of data.[28]

The value of these monitors becomes especially evident in two common situations. The first situation arises when clinicians or researchers consider whether a drug provides effective blood pressure control throughout the entire day.[42] For example, Floras's group[13] used these monitors to demonstrate that only two of four

FIGURE 6.5 Rate and Severity of Target Organ Damage in 108 Patients

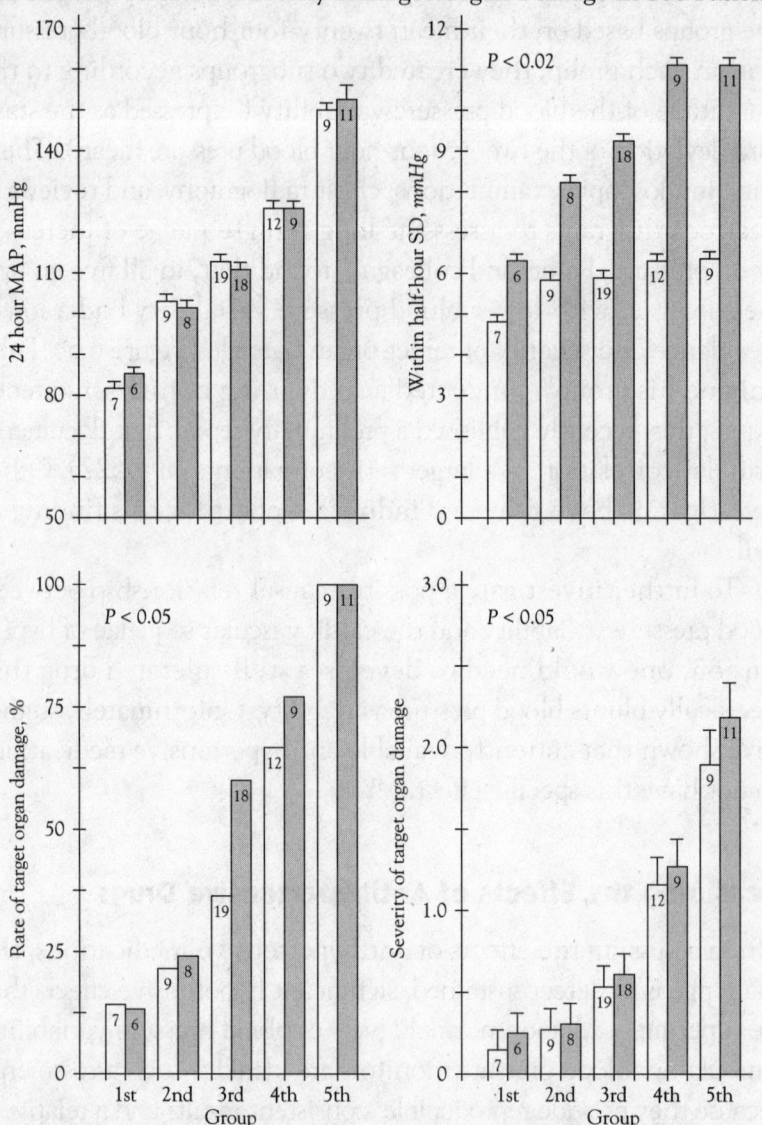

Note: Graph bars are for subgroups whose short-term blood pressure variability, expressed as within half-hour standard deviation of MAP, was below (~) or above (~) the average short-term variability of the group. Within each group, the two subgroups had a similar twenty-four-hour MAP, but the rate and severity of target organ damage was less in the group in which blood pressure variability was lower.

Source: From Parati, G., Pimidossi, G., Albini, F., Malaspina, D., & Mancia, G. (1987). Relationship of 24-hour blood pressure mean and variability to severity of target-organ damage in hypertension. *Journal of Hypertension, 5,* p. 97. Reprinted by permission.

antihypertensive agents belonging to the beta-blocker family (atenolol and long-acting propranolol) significantly reduced blood pressure throughout the entire twenty-four-hour period after dosing, despite the fact that all four of these drugs are used in a once-daily dosing schedule to control hypertension.

The second situation arises when determining a drug's peak and trough effects.[43] The *peak effect* is the maximal blood pressure reduction, and it generally occurs soon after dosing. The *trough effect* is the decrease in blood pressure seen just before administering the subsequent dose. Control of blood pressure at the trough is important, especially for once-daily drugs. Because these drugs traditionally are taken in the morning at breakfast, once-daily drugs may end up exposing patients to uncontrolled blood pressure in the early morning, just when blood pressure begins its normal diurnal rise and when cardiovascular risk is therefore the highest.

New Directions: Blood Pressure Variability in the Acute Care Setting

In summary, a now mature line of research has confirmed the existence of blood pressure variability and has characterized it in ambulatory, clinically stable patients. The research also suggests that information about this variability can be useful in the diagnosis of hypertension, assessment of its prognosis, and design of antihypertensive treatment strategies. As we refine our knowledge regarding blood pressure variability in the above setting, it is appropriate to consider whether such knowledge can be useful in entirely new settings, such as intensive care and perioperative care.

Rationale

Intensive and perioperative care are key components of our health care system. The technology-rich settings in which such care is rendered have come to symbolize both the strengths and weaknesses of modern medicine. Many of the most impressive breakthroughs involve intensive or perioperative care in some way, yet the care rendered in such settings is enormously expensive and sometimes viewed as excessive or, frankly, inappropriate.

Patients requiring intensive or perioperative care would be expected to have a large blood pressure variability. An underlying condition that necessitates acute care almost certainly causes major failings in the body's ability to exert homeostatic control over blood pressure and other physiological parameters. In the intensive care setting, for example, important and rapidly evolving blood pressure changes are part of common clinical syndromes, such as acute myocardial infarction and septic shock. In the operating room and postanesthesia recovery unit, blood loss and other fluid shifts also can have profound effects on blood pressure. Patients in both settings have an additional source of blood pressure variability: they often receive drugs and interventions that affect the cardiovascular system and blood pressure itself. Thus, in addition to normal physiological causes of blood pressure variability, acute care patients may have supervening causes for that variation.

The clinical recognition of and appropriate response to blood pressure changes may have more immediate importance for acute care patients than for ambulatory, clinically stable patients who were the subjects of the previous discussion. Indeed, it is easy to imagine situations in which the recognition of and appropriate response to blood pressure changes could have life-or-death implications.

Not surprisingly, virtually all patients in such acute settings receive frequent blood pressure checks, and a substantial proportion are monitored continuously through the use of intra-arterial catheter/pressure transducer systems. As a result, enormous amounts of data regarding blood pressure are available (or potentially available) for these patients. From a statistical viewpoint, this is a data-rich environment; and powerful statistical methods may be used in this type of environment to transform the data into clinically important information.

Ironically, despite a logical need to manage blood pressure with great precision in such acute settings and despite the great opportunity to do so afforded by the availability of so much data on blood pressure, the existing paradigms for blood pressure management in intensive and perioperative care settings do not account for blood pressure variability with anywhere near the degree of sophistication approached in the research reviewed above.

In fact, the current approach seems remarkably unassuming by comparison: physicians set limits for an uppermost and lowermost acceptable blood pressure, given the particulars of the case at hand; they instruct the nurses to notify them when the patient's blood pressure exceeds these limits; and when the care plan requires that blood pressure be continuously monitored, nurses program the monitoring system to sound an alarm when it senses that the physician's preset limits have been exceeded. In effect, this approach filters out most data about blood pressure variability except for the most extreme deviations.

The problem with this approach is that it discards information that may contribute to optimal patient care. Blood pressure that hovers just below a preset limit for extended periods of time may have more pathophysiological significance than a short run of observations in which a limit has been exceeded. Conversely, ascribing proper importance to a short string of observations in which a limit has been exceeded requires knowledge of preceding and ongoing observations. Furthermore, the act of filtering out data about blood pressure variabilities can impede recognition of trends in blood pressure, which are manifestations of the cardiovascular response to illness or to the perioperative state. Using computerized statistical methods to examine such trends in real time might enable providers to more quickly recognize changing clinical conditions. This use would be consistent with most clinicians' preferences to engage in preventive practices when possible.

Making use of all available patient-related blood pressure information may be important for other reasons as well. This information may enhance the understanding of acute diseases and of the perioperative state itself. Improved information on blood pressure thus may prove useful when predicting the clinical course, designing care plans, or predicting physiological stability and consequent readiness for discharge (from an intensive care unit or from the hospital). Alternatively, thorough and correctly interpreted information on blood pressure variability may effectively replace information currently obtained from expensive or risky diagnostic tests (for example, cardiac output, pulmonary wedge pressure).

Thus, the case for studying blood pressure variability in acute care settings can be summarized as follows. First, one can build from an already impressive knowledge base about blood pressure variability in other settings. Second, in the data-rich environments of intensive care and perioperative care units—environments that rival those of the most sophisticated research studies on this subject—data on blood pressure variability are already being collected. Third, it is reasonably likely that closer scrutiny of such blood pressure data will provide helpful insights for patient care.

Barriers to the Use of Data on Blood Pressure Variability in Acute Care

Before deciding whether to embark on this new line of research and selecting the specific research questions that should be posed, it is important to consider the substantial challenges associated with changing current care practices to accommodate new approaches to blood pressure variability. There are two potential barriers in this regard. First, the effort to obtain and analyze information on blood pressure variability might entail intolerable amounts of new work for providers. Second, it might increase the costs of acute care at a time when national attention is focused on the control of such costs.

More Work?   Clinicians in intensive and perioperative care settings already feel besieged by their workloads: enormous amounts of data, tremendous time pressure, and the constantly changing clinical challenges presented by the patients for whom they care are all components of this charged environment. They often work in cramped patient care areas, surrounded by catheters, tubes, monitors, and often electronic devices that are employed to treat these patients. They are faced with time-consuming demands to document patient-related information and to communicate with the many individuals involved in the care of each patient.

For an average post-operative patient, the ICU nurse may collect and record fifteen to one hundred data elements per hour. He or she collects this information from multiple sources, which include his or her own physical findings, bedside monitors, and hospital laboratories. Many acute care nurses state they spend more than 50 percent of their time collecting and documenting patient-related data. The physician's challenge is equally daunting: he or she spends much time inserting the tubes and catheters that enable monitoring to take place, assimilating the data that are generated, and developing care plans based on these data. Physicians who care for such patients are, of course, usually responsible for many of them at any one time.

In this context, it is highly unlikely that acute caregivers can accept an additional burden of data collection, data analysis, or documentation—or even find the space to place new monitoring equipment—to support such proposed research. Consequently, any effort to introduce information on blood pressure variability into the acute care setting must be sensitive to these constraints.

Higher Costs? Intensive care and perioperative care are particularly expensive components of a health care system that, by most accounts, already costs too much. The expenses associated with acute care are driven by the technologies housed within these acute care units and by the specialized personnel who operate these technologies. It would be imprudent to consider disseminating a new technology unless there was good reason to believe it would be cost-effective.

The Opportunity

The nature of the acute care patient, the complex work environment clinicians face when caring for such patients, and the societal requirement that new technologies add value to existing care all combine to create a challenging set of specifications for a new technology that could incorporate information about blood pressure variability into the provision of acute care. The new technology must record blood pressure noninvasively, analyze its variability in real time, and display the information in a form that is easily interpretable. Furthermore, it must be associated with little or no incremental cost increases and preferably reduce costs or foster care improvements when compared to current practice.

Remarkably, the technology is at hand to record, analyze, and display blood pressure-related information in real time. Until recently, intra-arterial techniques were required in order to continuously record information on blood pressure. Recently, however, an inexpensive bedside device, known as Finapres (Ohmeda Monitoring Systems, Englewood, Colorado), has become commercially available for this purpose. The device provides continual, noninvasive monitoring of blood pressure by using techniques based on the principle of vascular unloading and on a photoplethysmographic arterial/volume clamp method applied at the finger level.[44,45] Beat-to-beat blood pressure values obtained from this device are strongly correlated with those obtained simultaneously from an intra-arterial catheter.[45-47] This correlation persists during various maneuvers that cause sudden changes in blood pressure. Thus, the device appears to effectively follow trends in blood pressure. Some anesthesiologists already have begun to use this device for intraoperative blood pressure monitoring. The device is about the size of a bread box, and an even smaller, portable version has been developed.[48,49]

After noninvasively and inexpensively obtaining continuous information on blood pressure, the remaining technological challenge is to analyze and display blood pressure variability in real time. As mentioned above, this variability may be analyzed by many methods, and the selection of a method that balances the risk of information loss and unreliability with the need for a simple, easily understood calculation method becomes a critical issue.

Since Shewhart developed them more than sixty years ago[50], statisticians and engineers in many industries around the world have used *control charts* for this purpose. Today, evidence is overwhelming that these tools are simple to use while they offer profound insights about the data streams that arise from complex production processes, even as these processes continue to function. In other words, they provide real-time information about process performance.[51,52] Control charts would seem to be ideal tools to display and analyze data on blood pressure variability in acute care settings because they allow users to assimilate large amounts of patient-related data rapidly in a way that is statistically valid.

Some have speculated that control charts could be used as tools to assist clinical decision making[53-55], but to date, no one has published examples of types of use in mainstream clinical care. For three reasons, these tools have not yet had the profound effect on clinical care that they have in so many other settings outside health care. First, control charts are most useful in data-rich environments, ones in which it is possible to collect at least a few dozen observations inexpensively and during a reasonably short period of time. Unfortunately, most primary care and outpatient settings do not provide this opportunity. Second, members of the medical community are not familiar with the statistical methods used to create control charts or with their analysis. Third, and particularly relevant to the acute care setting, microcomputer software that would permit real-time transformation and analysis of physiological data has not been available.

Zimmerman and his coworkers[56-58] have developed microcomputer software (Biomedical Quality Control Corporation of America, Mobile, Alabama) that enables electronic transfer of blood pressure data—obtained from either intra-arterial catheter/transducer systems or noninvasive systems—from most acute care monitors into a personal computer. Once this has been accomplished, the computer software can (1) display, on screen or on hard copy in the form of a run chart, several hundred serially recorded sets of blood pressure recordings from an individual patient; (2) calculate in real time the mean and standard deviation of the mean for previously entered values; and (3) use the above to display the data in the form of X-bar and standard deviation charts.

The software can, in fact, simultaneously analyze and display up to four physiological variables, including blood pressure, heart rate, oxygen saturation, temperature, and central venous pressure. In addition, its graphical displays are easy to understand. Preliminary, off-line studies using this technology in burn units, sleep labs, and operating rooms have identified runs, jumps, cycles, and trends in a variety of patient groups[56-60], although such information has yet to be used by clinicians in real time.

The technologies described above are associated with low incremental costs, but their abilities to foster cost savings or care improvements are unclear at the present time. There is a reasonable possibility, however, that these technologies can improve the value of acute care. The two most important ways in which statistically valid, real-time analyses of blood pressure and blood pressure variability might improve the value of acute care are as follows:

1. *They can reduce the incidence of tampering.* Tampering is a phenomenon in which caregivers prescribe a new drug, change the dose of a drug, order additional tests, or intervene in some other way because they have incorrectly assumed that the patient's condition has changed, when in fact the patient is "stable." Tampering occurs when caregivers misinterpret the variation in serial recordings of a physiological variable such as blood pressure. Tampering increases direct costs due to inappropriate use of resources (waste), and it may be associated with increased indirect costs due to prolonged lengths of stay, drug side effects, and higher personnel costs as well. The actual incidence of tampering is unknown.

2. *They can improve the timeliness with which appropriate interventions are prescribed.* Subtle trends in blood pressure or changes in blood pressure variability itself (or similar changes in the other physiological parameters that can be tracked by using the same technology) can signal the clinically significant

events long before traditional "alarm limits" have been crossed. More timely interventions may reduce length of stay and the indirect costs of care.

Conclusion

Recent technological advances have given us an opportunity to expand the mature line of research on blood pressure variability into an entirely new clinical arena: acute care. Possibly, this expansion will enable us to improve the value of acute care. To undertake such an effort, however, two major hurdles need to be overcome. First, we have not trained health care professionals to apply statistically valid approaches to the assessment of individual patient variability. Second, we do not yet fully understand how to interpret blood pressure variability in acute care settings. At this point, both seem to be worthy challenges.

Notes

1. Hales, S. (1733). *Statistical essays* (Vol. 2). (W. Innys & R. Maubry, Eds.). London: Haemastaticks.

2. Bevan, A. T., Honour, A. J., & Stott, F. H. (1969). Direct arterial pressure recording in unrestricted man. *Clinical Science, 36,* 329–344.

3. Floras, J. S., Hassan, M. O., Jones, J. V., et al. (1988). Factors influencing blood pressure and heart rate variability in hypertensive humans. *Hypertension, 11,* 273–281.

4. Floras, J. S. (1981). *Studies on the neural regulation of blood pressure in hypertension.* Unpublished doctoral dissertation, University of Oxford, Oxford, England.

5. Mancia, G., & Zanchetti, A. (1986). Blood pressure variability. In A. Zanchetti & R. C. Tarazi (Eds.), *Handbook of hypertension: Vol. 7. Pathophysiology of hypertension-cardiovascular aspects* (pp. 125–152). Amsterdam: Elsevier.

6. Floras, J. S., Jones, J. V., Hassan, M. P., et al. (1981). Cuff and

ambulatory blood pressure in subjects with essential hypertension. *Lancet, 2,* 107–109.

7. Pickering, T. G., James, G. D., Boddi, C., et al. (1988). How common is white coat hypertension? *Journal of the American Medical Association, 259,* 225–228.

8. Pickering, T. G. (1987). Strategies for the evaluation and treatment of hypertension and some implications of blood pressure variability. *Circulation, 76*(Suppl. 1), 177–182.

9. Perloff, D., Sokolow, M., & Cowan, R. (1983). The prognostic value of ambulatory blood pressures. *Journal of the American Medical Association, 249,* 2792–2798.

10. Parati, G., Pomidossi, G., Albini, F., Malaspina, D., & Mancia, G. (1987). Relationship of 24-hour blood pressure mean and variability to severity of target-organ damage in hypertension. *Journal of Hypertension, 5,* 93–98.

11. Floras, J. S. (1991). Will knowing the variability of ambulatory blood pressure improve clinical outcome? *Clinical Investigations in Medicine, 14,* 231–240.

12. Watson, R.D.S., Lumb, R., Young, M. A., et al. (1987). Variation in cuff blood pressure in untreated outpatients with mild hypertension. *Journal of Hypertension, 5,* 207–211.

13. Floras, J. S., Hassan, M. O., Jones, J. V., & Sleight, P. (1983). Ambulatory blood pressure and its variability during randomized double-blind administration of atenolol, metoprolol, pindolol, and long-acting propranolol in subjects with mild to moderate hypertension. *Drugs, 25*(Suppl. 1), 19–25.

14. Di Rienzo, M., Grassi, G., Pedotti, A., & Mancia, G. (1983). Continuous vs. intermittent blood pressure measurements in estimating 24-hour average blood pressure. *Hypertension, 5,* 264–269.

15. Floras, J. S., Hassan, M. O., Jones, J. V., & Sleight, P. (1987). Pressor responses to laboratory stresses and daytime blood pressure variability. *Journal of Hypertension, 5,* 715–719.

16. Schauchinger, H., Langewitz, W., Schmieder, R., & Ruddel, H. (1989). Comparison of parameters for assessing blood pressure and heart rate variability from non-invasive twenty-four-hour blood pressure monitoring. *Journal of Hypertension, 7*(Suppl. 3), S81–S84.

17. Di Rienzo, M., Castiglioni, P., Mancia, G., et al. (1989). 24-hour sequential spectral analysis of arterial blood pressure and pulse interval in free-moving subjects. *IEEE Transactions on Biomedical Engineering, 36,* 1066–1075.

18. Littler, W. A., & Komsuoglu, B. (1989). Which is the most accurate method of measuring blood pressure? *American Heart Journal, 117,* 723–728.

19. Floras, J. S., Hassan, M. O., Jones, J. V., et al. (1988). Consequences of impaired arterial baroreflex in essential hypertension: Effects on pressor responses, plasma noradrenaline, and blood pressure variability. *Journal of Hypertension, 6,* 525–535.

20. Conway, J., Boon, N., Davies, C., et al. (1990). Neural and humoral mechanisms involved in blood pressure variability. *Journal of Hypertension, 2,* 203–208.

21. Van den Mairacker, A. H., Man In't Veld, A. J., Jan Eck, H.J.R., et al. (1987). Effects of bedrest and sensory deprivation on arterial pressure and heart rate variability in hypertensive man. *Journal of Hypertension, 5*(Suppl. 5), S475–S477.

22. Drummond, P. H. (1990). Parasympathetic cardiac control in mild hypertension. *Journal of Hypertension, 8,* 383–387.

23. Raftery, E. P., & Ward, A. P. (1968). The indirect method of recording blood pressure. *Cardiovascular Research, 2,* 210–218.

24. Mancia, G., Bertinieri, G., Grassi, G., et al. (1983). Effects of blood pressure measurement by the doctor on patients' blood pressure and heart rate. *Lancet, 2,* 695–697.

25. Ayman, D., & Goldshine, A. D. (1940). Blood pressure determinations by patients with essential hypertension: 1. The difference between clinic and home readings before treatment. *American Journal of Medical Science, 200,* 465–474.

26. White, W. B., Lund-Johansen, P., & Omvik, P. (1990). Assessment of four ambulatory blood pressure monitors and measurements by clinicians vs. intra-arterial blood pressure at rest and during exercise. *American Journal of Cardiology, 65,* 60–66.

27. Borkowski, K. R. (1989). The diagnosis and treatment of hypertension: Does ambulatory pressure monitoring have a role? *Canadian Medical Association Journal, 141,* 517–519.

28. Conway, J., Johnston, J., Coats, A., et al. (1988). The use of ambulatory blood pressure monitoring to improve the accuracy and reduce the numbers of subjects in clinical trials of antihypertensive agents. *Journal of Hypertension*, 6, 111–116.

29. Ruddy, M. C., Bialy, G. B., Malka, E. S., et al. (1988). The relationship of plasma renin activity to clinic and ambulatory blood pressure in elderly people with isolated systolic hypertension. *Journal of Hypertension*, 6(Suppl. 4), S412–S415.

30. Mancia, G., Parati, G., Albini, F., & Villani, A. (1988). Circadian blood pressure variations and their impact on disease. *Journal of Cardiovascular Pharmacology*, 12(Suppl. 7), S11–S17.

31. Weber, M. A. (1987). Cardiovascular outcomes of treating high blood pressure. *American Heart Journal*, 114, 964–971.

32. White, W. B. (1991). Ambulatory blood pressure and target organ involvement in hypertension. *Clinical Investigations in Medicine*, 14(3), 224–230.

33. Parati, G., Pomidossi, G., Albini, F., et al. (1987). Relationship of 24-hour blood pressure mean and variability to severity of target-organ damage in hypertension. *Journal of Hypertension*, 5, 93–98.

34. Pessina, A. C., Palatini, P., Sperti, G., et al. (1985). Evaluation of hypertension and related target organ damage by average day-time blood pressure. *Clinical Experiments in Hypertension*, [A]7, 267–278.

35. Palatini, P., Martina, S., Businaro, R., et al. (1990). Night time blood pressure (BP) and BP variability vs. cardiovascular complications in hypertension [Abstract]. *Journal of Hypertension*, 8(Suppl. 3), S89.

36. White, W. B., Dey, H. M., & Schulman, P. (1989). Assessment of the daily blood pressure load as a determinant of cardiac function in patients with mild to moderate hypertension. *American Heart Journal*, 118, 782–795.

37. Wilhelmsen, L., Berglund, G., Elmfeldt, E., et al. (1986). The multifactor primary prevention trial in Goteborg. *European Heart Journal*, 7, 279–288.

38. Pickering, T. G., Harshfield, G. A., Kleinert, H. D., et al. (1982). Blood pressure during normal daily activities, sleep, and exercise:

Comparison of values in normal and hypertensive subjects. *Journal of the American Medical Association, 247,* 992–996.

39. Clement, D. L., De Pue, N. Y., & Packet, L. (1987). Effect of calcium antagonists on ambulatory blood pressure and its variations. *Journal of Cardiovascular Pharmacology, 10*(Suppl. 3), S117–S119.

40. Novo, S., Alaimo, G., Giordano, U., et al. (1987). Ketanserin vs. propranolol in the treatment of mild and moderate essential hypertension: Corroboration with ambulatory blood pressure monitoring. *Journal of Cardiovascular Pharmacology, 10*(Suppl. 3), S104–S106.

41. Dupont, A. G., Vanderniepen, P., & Six, R. O. (1987). Effect of guanfacine on ambulatory blood pressure and its variability in elderly patients with essential hypertension. *British Journal of Clinical Pharmacology, 23,* 397–401.

42. Cheung, D. C., Gasster, J. L., & Weber, M. A. (1989). Assessing the duration of the antihypertensive effect with whole-day automated blood pressure monitoring. *Archives of Internal Medicine, 149,* 2021–2025.

43. Neutel, J. M., Schnaper, H., Cheung, D. G., et al. (1990). Antihypertensive effects of beta blockers administered once daily: 24-hour measurements. *American Heart Journal, 20,* 166–171.

44. Pena, J. (1973). Photoelectric measurement of blood pressure, volume, and flow in the finger. In *Digest of the International Conference on Medicine and Biological Engineering* (p. 104). Conference Committee of the 10th International Conference on Medicine and Biological Engineering, Dresden.

45. Wesseling, K. H., De Wit, B., Settles, J. J., & Klaver, W. H. (1982). On the indirect registration of finger blood pressure after Penaz. *Funkt Biol Medicine, 1,* 245–250.

46. Parati, G., Casadei, R., Groppellin, A., Di Rienzo, M., & Mancia, G. (1989). Comparison of finger and intra-arterial blood pressure monitoring at rest and during laboratory testing. *Hypertension, 13,* 647–655.

47. Imholz, B.P.M., Van Montfrans, G. A., Settels, J. J., et al. (1988). Continuous non-invasive blood pressure monitoring: Reliability of Finapres device during the Valsalva maneuver. *Cardiovascular Research, 22,* 390–397.

48. Idema, R. N., Van Der Meiracker, A. H., Imholz, B.P.M., et al. (1989). Comparison of Finapres non-invasive beat-to-beat finger blood pressures with intrabrachial artery pressures during and after bicycle ergometry. *Journal of Hypertension, 7*(Suppl. 6), 58–59.

49. Langewouters, G. J., De Wit, B., Van Der Hoeven, G.M.A., et al. (1990). Feasibility of continuous non-invasive 24-hour ambulatory measurement of finger arterial blood pressure with Portapres [Abstract]. *Journal of Hypertension, 8*(Suppl. 3), S88.

50. Shewhart, W. A. (1980). *Economic control of quality of manufactured product*. New York, NY: American Society for Quality Control. (Original work published 1931)

51. Grant, E. L., & Leavenworth, R. S. (1988). *Statistical quality control*. New York: McGraw-Hill.

52. Plsek, P. (1992). Introduction to control charts. *Quality Management in Health Care, 1*, 65–74.

53. Laffel, G., & Blumenthal, D. (1989). The case for using industrial quality management science in health care organizations. *Journal of the American Medical Association, 262*, 2869–2873.

54. Kritchevsky, S. B., & Simmons, B. P. (1992). Continuous quality improvement: Concepts and applications for physician care. *Journal of the American Medical Association, 266*, 1817–1823.

55. Blumenthal, D. (1993). Total quality management and physician's clinical decisions. *Journal of the American Medical Association, 269*, 2775–2778.

56. Zimmerman, S. M., Brown, L., Brown, S., & Alexander, L. (1990). Human body function control charts for the physician. *44th Annual Quality Congress Proceedings: American Society for Quality Control*, p. 118.

57. Zimmerman, S. M., Brown, L., Brown, S., & Goldhamer, R. L. (1990). Quality control charts: Analysis of patient data. *Eighth International Conference of the Israel Society for Quality Assurance Transactions*, pp. 8–18.

58. Zimmerman, S. M., Brown, L., Brown, S., & Zimmerman, R. (1992). Using the theory of runs in a biomedical application. *46th Annual Quality Congress Proceedings: American Society for Quality Control*, p. 23.

59. Zimmerman, S. M., & Brown, L. (1992). Using moving average process control charts in biomedical applications. *Ninth International Conference of the Israel Society for Quality Assurance Transactions*, pp. 18–23.

60. Zimmerman, S. M., Zimmerman, R., & Schoen, L. (1993). SPC analysis of patients: Sleep laboratory data. *American Statistical Association Conference Proceedings*, p. 77.

7

What Is TURP?

Controlling Variation in the Performance of Clinical Processes

Brent C. James, M.D., M.Stat.

Practice variation within Western health care delivery is a well-established fact. In 1938, Glover[1] demonstrated differences in the rates of tonsillectomy among various regions of England, beyond what could be explained by population differences. Three decades later, Lewis[2] found similar variation among surgical procedure rates in the United States. During the 1970s and 1980s, Wennberg and coworkers developed small area variation analysis (SAVA), a set of formal techniques for comparing hospitalization rates across small geographical areas. SAVA showed that American hospital admissions for some surgical procedures and medical diagnoses occurred at much higher rates in some communities than in other similar communities even after controlling for underlying population factors.[3] When comparing use rates for a group of surgical procedures and medical diagnoses among the United States, England, and Norway, McPherson and coworkers found that some showed consistently low ranges of variation within all three countries, whereas others showed consistently high ranges of variation across the three countries. This range of intercommunity variation was related to specific surgical procedures and medical diagnoses and was true even though the average use rates for each procedure or diagnosis varied significantly among the countries included in the study.

Chassin and coworkers[7] extended Wennberg's SAVA techniques to large geographical areas within the United States and confirmed similar high rates of variation. A team of researchers at Rand Corporation hypothesized that differences among communities could be explained by higher rates of inappropriate treatment in communities with high use rates. The RAND team developed formal methods to generate measurable indicators for several surgical procedures and medical hospitalizations[8] and then used those methods to assess several high-variation surgical procedures, medical procedures, and hospital admissions for medical diagnoses. They discovered that high-use rates were not consistently associated with high rates of inappropriate procedures and hospitalizations,[9,10] as they measured appropriateness.

Wennberg's SAVA and the RAND team's measures of appropriateness addressed a single class of issues: both examined the decision to treat a patient. Eddy[11] classified such decisions as *practice policies* and contrasted them with *performance policies*, which describe the manner in which a specified treatment or procedure is actually performed after the decision to treat has been made. Mulley makes an analogous distinction (see Chapter Four) between choosing the right thing to do (decision quality) and doing the right thing right (performance quality). Most variation studies have compared the use of medical services across populations of patients. These constitute in effect studies of variation in practice policies (Eddy's term) that reflect on quality of decision-making practices (decision quality) among geographically dispersed populations of doctors and patients. In contrast, studies of variation in performance policies (bearing on performance quality in Mulley's terminology) are relatively rare.

Henke and Epstein[12] examined differences among rheumatologists as they cared for patients with rheumatoid arthritis in an outpatient setting. Sage, Kessler, Sommers, and Silverman[13] noted differences among physicians when performing transurethral prostatectomies but provided only summary data on many of the factors involved in such care delivery. Other researchers have concentrated on exploring differences in the use rates of specific diagnostic tests across large groups of disparate patients (for example, within a department of internal medicine), but few studies compare individual physicians at a detailed level for specific treatments or diagnoses across a group of comparable patients.[14,15]

Given this body of existing research, investigators at Intermountain Health Care Institute decided to examine the manner of treatment (performance policies) at a detailed level across a group of physicians. To make fair comparisons, we selected a balanced cohort of similar patients, all diagnosed as suffering from symptomatic benign prostatic hypertrophy (BPH) without serious comorbidities at the time of hospital admission, who were treated with transurethral prostatectomy (TURP) and who did not receive major concurrent treatments during the same hospital admission. We chose TURP because it is a common procedure that has been shown to exhibit high variation in several SAVA studies, and it has been the focus of many studies that explore variation in the decision to treat. We hypothesized that we would find large differences among physicians' performance of TURP, similar to those already demonstrated by SAVA regarding the decision to use TURP to treat BPH in the first place. Such a finding could have important implications for in-hospital case management, outcomes research, the generation of practice guidelines, and public health policy development regarding quality and cost controls.

Methods

Intermountain Health Care (IHC) is a system of twenty-four hospitals located in Utah and southeastern Idaho that supply about 50 to 60 percent of all hospital-based health care delivered in the region. All use a single cost-based financial data system and contribute audited summary financial/clinical records to a centralized case-mix database for every inpatient or outpatient encounter. The financial system routinely tracks clinical care delivery at a detailed level for all billable items or activities. For example, it records each laboratory test, by type; each imaging examination, by type; each dose of a drug administered to a patient, by dose and specific drug; hours on an acute care nursing floor, adjusted for nursing acuity; and total minutes in a surgical suite. Costs for each individual item are computed from time and motion studies of personnel time, supplemented by direct measures of materials costs, amortized equipment costs, space allocations based on physical space use and amortized building and maintenance costs, and proportional assignment of administrative overhead.

We drew patients from all four large, community-based, acute care IHC hospitals (with 520, 389, 380, and 243 licensed beds) that serve Utah's Wasatch Front (including Ogden, Salt Lake City, and Provo, Utah). These hospitals serve similar urban communities within a limited geographical area. At the time of the study, all four hospitals offered a similar range of urologic services to their patients. One hospital sponsored a urologic residency training program with instruction provided by the community physicians who formed the hospital's urologic staff. Urology services at the remaining three institutions were staffed exclusively by community-based private urologists.

To select those patients who were potentially eligible for inclusion in the study, we used the final discharge assignment of DRG 336 (transurethral prostatectomy) for all cases admitted during 1985. Of the four hospitals in the study, the two smallest hospitals had relatively low patient volumes, compared with their larger counterparts. Therefore, we added cases from the last half of 1984 for those two facilities in order to increase their case volumes for the study, working backward from the end of the 1984 year. On the basis of ICD-9 diagnosis and procedure discharge codes included in the computerized records, we eliminated cases that did not have a primary diagnosis of BPH or that had received a major concurrent procedure that could bias measurement of patterns of care.

We planned to use the detailed financial record to track many of the specific characteristics of patients and their care but realized that not all important clinical decisions were reflected as billable items. We therefore formed a team of senior urologists and urology nurses representing the four participating hospitals. This group prepared lists of potential admission comorbidities that could change a patient's care; in-hospital complications that could change a patient's care; and important clinical factors that affected performance decisions but were not reflected in the financial system. These factors were used to build a standardized chart review form. We prepared lists of potential comorbidities and complications so that the chart review team could examine each patient record for specific factors, rather than depend on spontaneous recognition of possible comorbidities and complications during chart review.

Between the computerized financial system and the manual chart review, we tracked the following indicators of how each patient's care was performed: clinical laboratory (number of each specific test performed for each patient); microbiology laboratory (number of each specific type of culture or culture and sensitivity performed for each patient); pharmacy (type, dose, and number of doses for each drug used for each patient); imaging (type and number of each radiographic, MRI, or ultrasound examination performed for each patient); blood bank (number and type of each blood product preparation order and the amount and type of blood products actually transfused for each patient); central supply (dollar amount of supplies charged to each patient); weight of prostatic tissue removed at surgery, as reported by pathology; Foley catheter management (type of Foley catheter employed, irrigation schedule and type of irrigation, and whether the patient was recatheterized after initial removal of the Foley catheter, to relieve acute obstruction); and specific timings (time of admission, time of entry to operating room, time of anesthesia induction, procedure start time, procedure end time, time of entry to recovery room, time of return to nursing care floor, time of initial removal of Foley catheter, and time of discharge). All times were recorded as dates and clock times, so it was possible to calculate timings to the level of hours or minutes. With regard to all performance factors, we tracked only those activities that occurred within the hospital.

Using the standardized chart review form, three senior quality assurance nurses and two financial analysts jointly reviewed the medical records for all cases coded as DRG 336 (transurethral prostatectomy). The team individually classified each comorbidity and in-hospital complication by using a four-level staging system:

Blank.   Comorbidity or complication not present in record

Stage 0: Insignificant, requiring little or no modifications to care

Stage 1: Minor, requiring some modifications to care

Stage 2: Serious, requiring significant modifications to care

Stage 3: Life threatening, requiring major modifications to care

In the case of blood loss (the most common complication observed on the study), the four-level staging system was modified:

Blank: No blood loss recorded

Stage 0: Insignificant—"red-tinged urine"

Stage 1: Minor—"grossly bloody urine"

Stage 2: Major—up to four units of blood transfused

Stage 3: Serious—major bleeding episode with very difficult control, requiring more than four units of blood transfusions in the immediate postoperative period

All classifications were made by the consensus of the team after review by all members of the team. In the course of examining the patient records, the review team also added a small number of comorbidities and complications to the lists originally generated by the clinical oversight group. We used the highest single score for any comorbidity and the highest single score for any complication to identify patients with significant comorbidities on admission or significant in-hospital complications associated with their treatment.

Principal long-term outcomes of TURP include symptom relief, incontinence, impotence, and death. We used our computerized case mix data systems to identify major treatment failures, defined as those patients who were readmitted to an IHC facility for treatment of urinary obstruction within one year of initial TURP surgery. Because the vast majority of these cases fell under the purview of the Medicare system, we used Medicare's record of death within thirty days of hospital discharge to track mortality. We had no adequate measures of incontinence or impotence.

Finally, we merged the computerized patient records (from the financial/clinical data system) with those data elements collected through chart review. Analysis proceeded in two stages. The first stage included all patient records and tested for associations among comorbidities, complications, and outcomes and specific patient, physician, or hospital performance factors. In the second stage, performance factors among physicians and hospitals were compared. For the second stage, we eliminated those patients with a highest admission comorbidity score of two or higher or a highest in-hospital complication score of two or higher on the basis that such comorbidities or complications could reasonably change the care process and bias comparisons of performance indicators.

All patient records used in the study listed codes for both an attending physician and a surgeon. In those few cases for which the attending physician and the surgeon were different practitioners (both were still urologists for all cases), we used the surgeon code when analyzing performance indicators specifically associated with surgery (for example, grams of prostatic tissue removed or surgical procedure time), but the attending code was used for all other indicators. When doing physician comparisons, we combined cases for physicians who performed only very small numbers of eligible TURPs (fewer than five cases during the study period) and analyzed them as a separate group. Of the sixteen physicians with sufficient patient volume to be analyzed separately, only one (with five cases) had fewer than ten eligible cases in the final performance comparison group.

For each indicator of performance, we used appropriate statistical tests (for example, ANOVA for continuous data or Pearson's chi-squared test for categorical data) to determine any statistically significant differences among the physicians or the hospitals under study. For each factor, we also calculated the mean, median, variance, and range by physician. We then selected the physician with the lowest and the physician with the highest mean and/or median value for that performance indicator. We used those two values to represent the range of physician performance across the group.

Results

Table 7.1 is a summary of case accrual and exclusions within the study. A diagnosis of carcinoma of the prostate, made as a result of the TURP itself, was by far the most common reason that cases were ruled ineligible (of 177 cases classified as "principal diagnosis not benign prostatic hypertrophy," 174 resulted from findings of prostatic carcinoma incidental to the TURP procedure). Subsequent analysis revealed that an incidental finding of prostatic carcinoma during a routine TURP did not change the care process for that particular hospitalization. The second most common cause of patient ineligibility was the performance of a major secondary surgical procedure (most commonly an inguinal herniorrhaphy). Hospital B showed a significantly higher rate of secondary surgical procedures than the other hospitals in the study ($p = 0.042$, chi-squared test). The difference was statistically significant ($p = 0.0015$, ANOVA) but small in mean patient age among the hospitals (74.2, 69.6, 72.0, and 68.4 years for Hospitals A, B, C, and D, respectively). Otherwise, no significant differences were found among hospitals or physicians in terms of presenting comorbidities or numbers of patients excluded from the study, by specific reasons.

Table 7.2 shows complications observed among all patients (before exclusions) following TURP. By far, the most common was blood loss requiring transfusion. The most common long-term treatment failure was urethral contractures requiring surgical correction

TABLE 7.1 Case Accrual. # cases (percent of hospital's total cases)

	Hospital				
	A	B	C	D	Total
DRG 336 (TURP) cases					
All 1985 cases	249	133	95	60	537
Last half 1984 cases	—	—	92	61	153
Total DRG 336 cases	249	133	187	121	690
Ineligible cases excluded					
Principal dx not BPH	69 (27.7%)	34 (25.6%)	40 (21.4%)	34 (28.1%)	177 (25.7%)
Major concurrent procedure	18 (7.2%)	15 (11.3%)	8 (4.3%)	8 (6.6%)	49 (7.1%)
Missing chart	12 (4.8%)	5 (3.8%)	13 (7.0%)	11 (9.1%)	41 (5.9%)
"Other"[a]	2 (0.8%)	—	—	1 (0.8%)	3 (0.4%)
Total ineligible cases	101 (40.6%)	54 (40.6%)	61 (32.6%)	54 (44.6%)	270 (39.1%)
Total eligible cases	148 (59.4%)	79 (59.4%)	126 (67.4%)	67 (55.4%)	420 (60.9%)
Cases analyzed separately					
Significant comorbidity	9 (3.6%)	12 (9.0%)	15 (8.0%)	12 (9.9%)	48 (7.0%)
Significant complication	10 (4.0%)	5 (3.8%)	6 (3.2%)	7 (5.8%)	28 (4.1%)
Low case volume physician	36 (14.5%)	—	26 (13.9%)	5 (4.1%)	67 (9.7%)
Total cases analyzed separately	55 (22.1%)	17 (12.8%)	47 (25.1%)	24 (19.8%)	143 (20.7%)
Total cases in variation analysis	93 (37.3%)	62 (46.6%)	79 (42.2%)	43 (35.5%)	277 (40.1%)

within one year of initial TURP surgery. Urethral contractures concentrated in Hospital A (odds ratio = 6.62, p = 0.019, Mantel-Haenszel chi-squared test). Contractures were significantly associated with low amounts of prostatic tissue removed (p = 0.016, Student's t test): a mean of 30.2 grams of prostatic tissue was removed from patients who did not go on to experience contractures, whereas a mean of only 13.2 grams of prostatic tissue was removed from those patients who did experience contractures (see Table 7.3). Grams of prostatic tissue removed showed a strong association with true surgical procedure time (p < 0.00001, OLS regression), but surgical procedure times did not show a statistically significant association with later occurrence of urethral contractures. Figure 7.1 shows median true surgical procedure times (in minutes) and median amount of prostatic tissue excised (in grams, as reported by pathology) for each surgeon in the study.

Table 7.4 is a summary of variation in major performance factors across the sixteen surgeons and four hospitals in the study. Variation among physicians was statistically significant (p < 0.01, ANOVA) for all factors examined. Table 7.4 focuses on only five elements among the much larger group of elements tracked. We chose to concentrate on the elements listed because they were critical components of the major outcomes associated with a TURP (including medical results and costs) and because there was some question whether an inpatient system could detect accurately all performance indicators for other elements of care (for example, inpatient measurement would have failed to detect laboratory testing or radiographic examinations that a physician ordered on an outpatient basis, before a patient was admitted to the hospital). However, every care element that we tracked showed similar, statistically significant ranges of variation across the physician group. Length of stay (LOS) was the primary determinant of total hospital cost for the hospitalization (adjusted R^2 = 73.2 percent, p < 0.0001, OLS regression). LOS was strongly associated with whether surgery was performed on the day of (mean LOS: 3.04 days) or the day following (mean LOS: 4.63 days) hospital admission (p <

TABLE 7.2 Complications, by Hospital. # cases (percent of hospital's total cases)

			Hospital		
	A	B	C	D	Total
Total cases	249	133	187	121	690
Inpatient complications					
Blood loss	21 (8.4%)	7 (5.3%)	24 (12.8%)	15 (12.4%)	67 (9.7%)
Urethral obstruction	2 (0.8%)	—	2 (1.1%)	—	4 (0.6%)
Fever or infection	2 (0.8%)	—	—	2 (1.7%)	4 (0.6%)
Thrombophlebitis	—	2 (5.1%)	—	1 (0.8%)	3 (0.4%)
Cardiac complications	—	1 (0.8%)	—	1 (0.8%)	2 (0.3%)
BP drop in recovery	—	2 (1.5%)	—	—	2 (0.3%)
Pulmonary complications	1 (0.4%)	—	—	1 (0.8%)	1 (0.1%)
Other - atonic bladder, incontinence, etc.	—	—	1 (0.5%)	(5.8%)	2 (0.3%)
Long-term complications					
Urethral contractures	7 (2.8%)	—	2 (1.1%)	—	9 (1.3%)
Total complications	33 (13.3%)	12 (9.0%)	29 (15.5%)	20 (16.5%)	94 (13.6%)
Patient readmitted within one year for reobstruction	11 (4.4%)	—	3 (1.6%)	2 (1.7%)	16 (2.3%)

TABLE 7.3 Mean Grams of Prostatic Tissue Excised, by Physician Group

Physician group	Number of physicians	Number of cases	Mean gram weight of tissue removed
Number cases w/contractures	9	160	31.82
1 case w/contractures	5	79	28.88
2 cases w/contractures	2	34	21.15

0.00001, Student's t test). Surgery on the day of hospital admission was not associated with patient comorbidity on presentation or with the distances a patient had to travel to reach the hospital. Foley catheter management also affected length of stay. Table 7.5 illustrates hospital timing differences for five selected surgeons.

Discussion

Wennberg and coworkers[4] and Eddy[16] argued persuasively that practice variation in American medicine results primarily from professional uncertainty regarding available treatments and their outcomes. Among other causes, professional uncertainty arises from a significant lack of valid information regarding the outcomes of common medical practices; delays in dissemination of the valid information available; human limitations when dealing with large volumes of complex information; differences in observation and measurement error; geographical differences in the type and availability of health care resources; and differences in patient values, preferences, understanding, and communication styles.[17] Professional uncertainty also can magnify variation arising from secondary causes, such as financial incentives.[4] These types of arguments led to the reasonable premise that better scientific information regarding the outcomes of common medical practices could reduce professional uncertainty and diminish practice variation. Anecdotal information suggested that as practice variation declined, medical

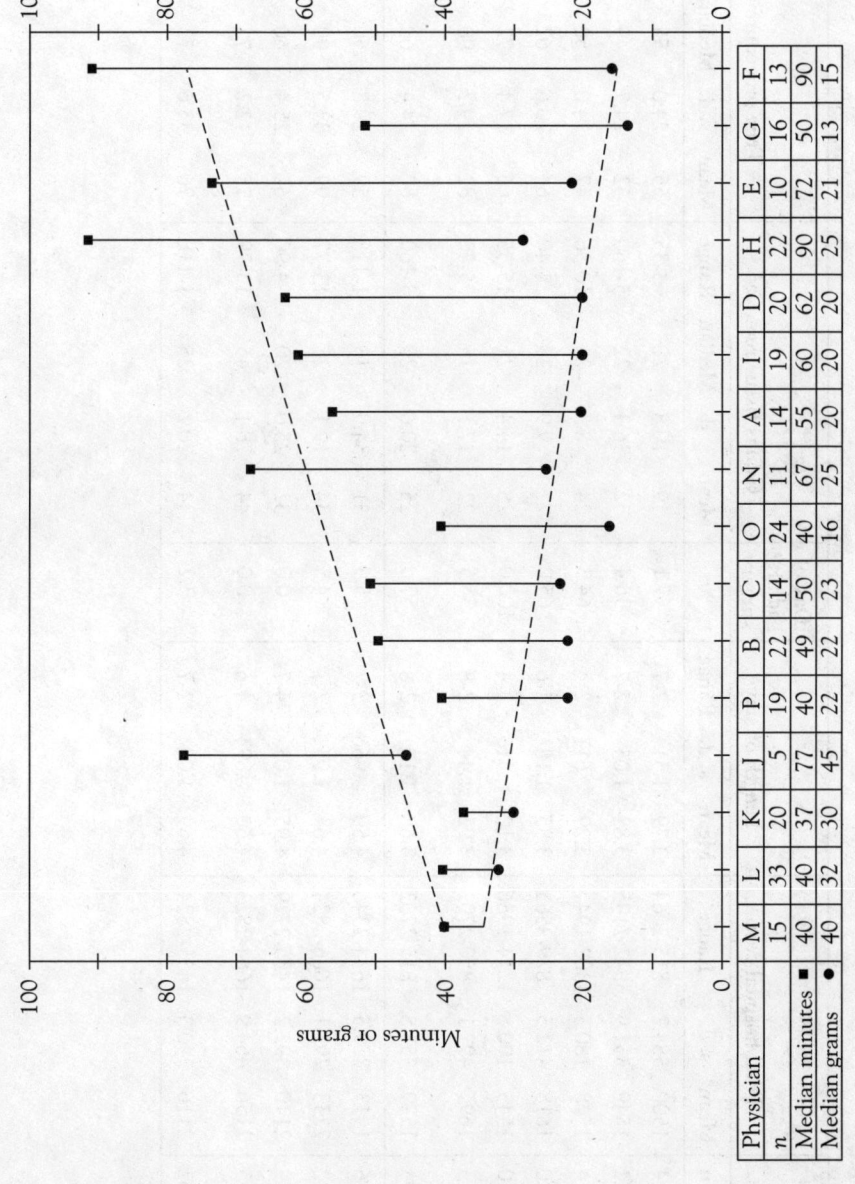

FIGURE 7.1 Median Procedure Time Versus Median Tissue Excised

Physician	M	L	K	J	P	B	C	O	N	A	I	D	H	E	G	F
n	15	33	20	5	19	22	14	24	11	14	19	20	22	10	16	13
Median minutes ■	40	40	37	77	40	49	50	40	67	55	60	62	90	72	50	90
Median grams ●	40	32	30	45	22	22	23	16	25	20	20	20	25	21	13	15

Minutes or grams

TABLE 7.4 Selected Hospital and Physician Performance Factors

Provider		Total hospital cost			Length of stay			Day of admit surgery	Grams tissue removed				True procedure time			
ID	n	Mean	s. d.	Range	Mean	s. d.	Range	%	Mean	s. d.	Median	Range	Mean	s. d.	Median	Range
A	14	1500	384.2	815-2064	3.79	1.31	2-7	57.1	19	10.8	20	3-35	55	24.0	55	25-110
B	22	1549	331.9	942-2195	3.82	1.05	2-7	36.4	32	36.3	22	5-160	52	24.7	49	20-135
C	14	1568	180.3	1302-1947	3.29	.611	2-4	64.3	24	8.3	23	10-36	47	14.0	50	25-65
D	20	1618	412.5	829-2565	3.85	1.18	2-6	65.0	22	9.9	20	4-40	64	20.6	62	20-105
E	10	1543	190.8	1214-1986	3.10	.316	3-4	100.0	28	14.4	21	15-55	66	17.4	72	25-80
F	13	1697	497.1	850-2702	3.92	1.44	2-8	38.5	22	17.1	15	5-70	82	29.2	90	35-120
Hosp A	93	1579	353.8	815-2702	3.68	1.10	2-8	57.0	25	20.6	20	3-160	60	24.4	60	20-135
G	16	1913	209.5	1634-2346	4.50	.966	3-7	5.9	31	34.9	13	1-118	59	29.8	50	20-137
H	22	2233	292.1	1666-2824	4.64	1.05	2-7	4.5	34	19.1	28	13-77	99	33.5	90	60-195
I	19	2140	392.2	1435-2729	4.95	1.03	4-7	0.0	32	25.0	20	4-90	62	25.4	60	22-102
J	5	2156	464.9	1664-2823	4.60	.894	4-6	0.0	44	28.1	45	13-79	75	12.2	77	58-90
Hosp B	62	2116	340.3	1435-2824	4.69	1.00	2-7	3.2	34	26.2	25	1-118	76	33.6	72	20-195

Provider		Total hospital cost			Length of stay			Day of admit surgery	Grams tissue removed				True procedure time			
ID	n	Mean	s.d.	Range	Mean	s.d.	Range	%	Mean	s.d.	Median	Range	Mean	s.d.	Median	Range
K	20	1598	295.3	1179-2302	4.60	1.27	3-8	22.2	32	21.8	30	10-85	45	19.5	37	20-89
L	33	1269	353.9	624-2355	3.21	1.17	1-6	66.7	39	29.9	32	5-115	43	19.8	40	15-90
M	15	1164	253.2	893-1797	2.73	1.03	2-5	80.0	42	24.6	40	5-80	43	16.9	40	20-77
N	11	1552	100.1	1402-1683	3.36	.505	3-4	90.9	32	20.8	25	12-75	69	20.7	67	30-97
Hosp C	79	1372	340.5	624-2355	3.49	1.28	1-8	62.3	37	25.7	30	5-115	48	20.9	43	15-97
O	24	1556	233.5	1045-2153	4.29	.955	3-7	20.8	18	12.8	16	4-59	40	14.3	40	20-70
P	19	1662	384.4	1130-2676	4.53	1.58	3-8	42.1	23	12.0	22	6-44	41	11.3	40	15-65
Hosp D	43	1603	309.9	1045-2676	4.40	1.26	3-8	30.2	20	12.6	16	4-59	41	13.0	15-70	15-70
All	277	1644	433.1	624-2824	3.96	1.25	1-8	42.2	30	23.4	23	1-160	57	27.4	27.4	15-195
Inter-MD range		1164-2233 (1.92x)			2.73-4.95 (1.81x)			0-100	Mean: 18-44 (2.44x) Median: 13-45 (3.46x)				Mean: 40-99 (2.48x) Median: 37-90 (2.43x)			

TABLE 7.5 Median Hospital Times for Five Selected Surgeons

Physician	Hours from admission to surgery	Hours from surgery to Foley removal	Recath rate (%)	Hours from Foley removal to discharge	Total hospital hours
1	5.33	46.08	0	14.54	65.95
2	18.86	48.55	6	26.85	94.26
3	7.42	24.71	33	25.13	52.26
4	20.25	42.17	20	27.29	89.71
5	2.33	47.09	0	25.88	75.30

outcomes would improve and health care costs would fall (for example, both goals can be achieved simultaneously by using better scientific information to significantly reduce unnecessary treatments). Recognition of professional uncertainty's role in contributing to practice variation, both in the decision to apply a treatment and in the manner in which a particular treatment is performed, highlights American medicine's pressing need for better scientific information regarding all aspects of care delivery.

The gold standard for generating valid clinical information is the randomized controlled clinical trial (RCT). In traditional use, RCTs test efficacy; they compare the outcomes of a new treatment with those of alternative treatments in a very carefully controlled environment that minimizes potential sources of bias that could cloud judgments of outcomes. To that end, they usually are restricted to tightly defined groups of matched patients, with the goal of eliminating recognized or unrecognized sources of potential bias (for example, Angell[18], in discussing the failure to include women in RCTs, notes that "all subjects in a clinical trial would ideally be identical"; they randomize treatment assignment to minimize the risk of unknown sources of potential bias; and they control care delivery through strict treatment protocols designed to eliminate bias that results from systematic variation in the treatments themselves. As currently implemented, most RCTs function as a separate coordination, control, and data-gathering system added to the routine care-delivery processes. As a result, RCTs suffer from two serious limitations. First, they are difficult to organize, expensive to conduct, and often require long periods for patient accrual. These factors significantly impede the ability of RCTs to meet, in a timely manner, the large and expanding need among health care providers for reliable scientific data to guide treatment. Second, because RCTs use highly selected patient groups to control potential bias, real questions arise regarding the generalizability of their results to the larger universe of patients who do not match every criterion used to select eligible patients for the original trial but who still need treatment.

Practical limitations of RCTs pose clear impediments to American medicine's obvious need for extensive, timely, valid scientific information regarding best treatment practices for routine patient care. In response, a number of investigators have advanced alternative study designs. Their proposals balance control of possible bias against generalizability of results in the context of a trial administration system that collects, centralizes, collates, and validates data, that controls care delivery, and that coordinates the study group.

Hospital Firms

In 1985, Neuhauser[19] proposed—and then demonstrated—that hospital firms provided a viable means to conduct RCTs while avoiding most of their pitfalls. The firm method establishes groups of parallel providers, each representing a different treatment arm to be compared in the study. Eligible patients are assigned randomly among the groups. Data collection and control of treatment protocols are integrated into the delivery of care. Consequently, the firm method achieves significant operational efficiencies when compared with traditional RCT management methods.

Hospital firms appear to work well when patients can be assigned randomly to parallel provider groups, as in resident clinics in an academic teaching center. Unfortunately, most American practice environments—the private practice of medicine in the community setting—do not provide parallel care delivery groups or allow random patient assignment among groups. The firm method provides an effective implementation strategy for many of the ideas that lie at the heart of quality improvement study design, such as iterative improvement and integrated data systems that simultaneously serve the needs of both case management and the generation of valid new knowledge in a setting of routine care.

Effectiveness (Outcomes) Research

Wennberg led those who proposed effectiveness research as a means to rapidly generate valid clinical knowledge regarding the outcomes of specific treatment strategies. Effectiveness research gives up careful control of potential biases to gain the opportunity to study day-to-day patient care, so the outcomes are from real patients as they receive routine treatment in real settings. To that end, Wennberg suggested that large databases (for example, databases generated from insurance claims, such as HCFA data on Medicare inpatient treatment) could generate valid clinical information to inform treatment decisions, reduce professional uncertainty, and control health care costs. He summarized his arguments in testimony to Congress in 1984.[5] Those arguments contributed directly to the formation of the federal Agency for Health Care Policy and Research (AHCPR), with a legislative mandate to perform outcomes research (realized as patient outcomes research teams, or PORTs) and to generate practice guidelines from PORT results, careful reviews of the existing scientific literature, and consensus panels of medical experts.[20] Wennberg and others published an example of his proposed outcomes research methods in 1989. That study used information drawn from health insurance databases to compare the outcomes of TURP for BPH with the outcomes obtained using open prostatectomy for the same condition. It found that TURP had a higher mortality rate than the alternative procedure.[21] A follow-up study conducted by Sidney and coworkers[22], using data from the northern California Kaiser-Permanente system, obtained similar results. Similar to Wennberg's approach, Elwood championed the development of an extended system for effectiveness analysis in the private sector and called for the creation of new databases that track and analyze patient outcomes across all health care providers and that capture information not generally available in existing large, national databases.[23]

Effectiveness research, especially when based on large existing databases designed primarily for other uses, has problems of its own. They fall into three general categories:

1. *Bias introduced by unequal patient selection.* In an editorial accompanying the original article by Roos and coworkers[21] comparing TURP with open prostatectomy, Greenfield[24] noted that patient differences among treatment groups could fatally bias the outcome comparisons produced in such studies. In 1992, Concato, Horowitz, Feinstein, Elmore, and Schiff[25] provided data suggesting that exactly this had happened in Roos's analysis—that by failing to control for patient risk factors, Roos's study overestimated TURP mortality rates and probably reached inaccurate conclusions.

2. *Bias introduced by variation in treatments.* A fundamental principle of clinical trial design is that to fairly compare outcomes of different treatments, it is essential that the treatments be performed in a consistent manner. Otherwise, it is impossible to determine whether differences in outcomes among treatments arise from the treatments themselves or from the differences introduced by treatment variation. For that reason, RCTs use strict treatment protocols to control treatment delivery and to eliminate potential sources of bias.

In most effectiveness studies, however, it is impossible to determine how treatments were performed. Within those studies, variation in treatment performance could introduce significant bias into outcome comparisons. For example, our results (reported in the preceding tables) clearly show that significant differences exist among practitioners in performance of TURP and that those differences relate directly to patient outcomes. In fact, differences were so large among urologic surgeons that it is not at all clear that the entity coded as a "TURP" in large administrative databases describes a single procedure. It may be very important to discover the best way to perform a TURP (in terms of patient outcomes) before concluding whether, when, and how TURPs should be employed.

3. *Ability to inform clinical practice.* Much effectiveness research (especially that branch represented by outcomes research) focuses on patient outcomes alone. But practitioners do not directly make decisions about outcomes. They make decisions about a process of care. Although outcomes measures are essential to evaluate the value of alternative practices, the occurrence of outcomes must be related to the providers' actual decisions and actions if those providers are to have a basis upon which to change practices. Berwick[26] asks: "How can the root causes of differences in results be discovered? This is the most significant question because [unless] there is a method to discover the reasons underlying the differences, knowledge of results is useful only for judgment, not for improvement. Information on results, alone, is simply not enough because knowing how well something works is different from knowing how it works."

Quality Improvement

A *process* is a series of linked, often (but not necessarily) sequential steps designed to cause some set of outcomes to occur. Essentially, all of organized health care delivery can be described as a series of interlinked processes. In fact, the idea aptly describes any repetitive human activity designed to cause a set of outcomes to occur, add value, or transform inputs into outputs. Shewhart[27] developed methods to manage and optimize processes in routine production settings. He was interested particularly in variation in process performance. He believed that data on variation in a process's steps and outcomes can show a great deal about the internal operation and possible optimization of that process.[28] Because Shewhart aimed to develop knowledge for improvement in routine settings, his resulting quality improvement (QI) theory contains both a management philosophy and a scientific methodology. Although the management philosophy dominates many discussions of QI, its scientific methodology has strong ties to traditional medical study designs.[29] Furthermore, Shewhart's insights and methods effectively counter the difficulties in traditional efficacy or effectiveness research.

As with the hospital firms methodology, QI methods integrate administrative control and data collection into the care process itself. QI methods generate data that are generalizable because they focus on ordinary patient groups in a routine setting. Finally, such methods attempt to control bias by direct process measurement and control in an iterative fashion by using the general tools that Shewhart developed for process management.

QI study designs rest on four major elements: (1) a cohort of similar patients, (2) a stable process of care, (3) a set of prioritized outcomes, and (4) an integrated measurement and analysis system.

Patient Cohorts (Indications for Treatment). QI patient cohorts are formed by using objective eligibility criteria. In general, the criteria seek to identify a group of patients who should receive the same process of care and achieve the same level of results (allowing for small variations introduced by random patient factors). Eligibility criteria tend to be less stringent than those found in traditional RCTs but are compatible with the method's application in routine treatment settings, a desire to ensure generalizability of results, and often a focus on existing treatment alternatives, rather than on completely new treatments. To control for variation in patient factors that may influence observed treatments and outcomes, severity of illness measures can be used.

Process Control (Performance Indicators). Within a traditional RCT, formal protocols eliminate variation in performance of care. In contrast, QI trials use an iterative feedback system to measure and control variation in performance over time. That means that QI studies proceed in two stages: the first stage concentrates on the measurement and elimination of practice variation; the second stage uses the resulting stability and consistency in process of care to facilitate rigorous comparisons of alternative treatment methods. In effect, QI process monitors are dynamic, ever-changing, but rigorous protocols; the clinical team defines and refines the care process iteratively, over time, as the team cares for real patients in a routine care delivery setting.

Outcomes. Clinical QI studies usually track three classes of outcomes: (1) medical outcomes, including patient perceptions; (2) patient satisfaction; and (3) cost of care, including estimates of costs resulting from untreated disease within patients' lives. Some studies add measures of employee and professional satisfaction. As with other study designs, a QI study very frequently will select a few high-priority outcomes from a more exhaustive list based on the specific goals of a particular investigation.

Measurement and Analysis. To develop measures of processes of care, QI starts with flowcharts that resemble practice guidelines.[17] The flowcharts help identify elements that must be measured to document patient selection, track performance factors, and follow outcomes. In most cases, QI follows routine care processes, so required data elements are often part of the standard clinical record. Therefore, with careful planning, it is often possible to integrate a quality measurement system into the care delivery process itself and to avoid the high overhead associated with independent, external measurement systems. When integrated into a care delivery process, QI measurement functions as detailed case management, further justifying its use in an operational setting.

In studying processes, Shewhart[27,28] distinguished between two types of variation. *Common causes* (which Deming later called *random variation*) represent the sum of many small factors that exist in any process. Every real process demonstrates a significant component of such variation that typically follows random statistical distribution theory. Because common causes represent the sum of many small factors, attempts to explain random deviations usually fail because the associated variance is spread among many contributing factors. For a clinical process, common cause variation includes the small differences within a patient cohort that slip through the relatively loose eligibility criteria required by a real-world care delivery system. Common causes represent *appropriate* variation; they are expected in any real care delivery process as clinicians react to differences in patient presentation and preferences.

Special causes (assignable variation) arise from external factors that are not part of the underlying routine system of care delivery. These factors can often be identified through diligent effort. Clinicians can identify and manage special causes by identifying outliers in performance or outcome measures, tracking such outliers to root causes and then, when appropriate, eliminating those causes.

Shewhart developed statistical process control (SPC) to help with the first step in that sequence, the identification of outliers: SPC is a probability function that separates common from special causes (or, alternatively, random from assignable variation; appropriate from inappropriate variation).[30,31] Shewhart also argued that graphs were far more effective than tables of numbers for quick and accurate interpretation of data.[32] Shewhart therefore emphasized graphical methods to display SPC data. As an example, Figures 7.2 to 7.6 show the same data summarized in Table 7.4, presented as SPC charts that, for each measurement factor, compare each surgeon to the weighted mean for the whole physician group. Ott and Shilling[31] noted that longitudinal data often convey far more information about a process's performance than do a series of unconnected snapshots of the same data.

Finally, QI's methods recognize that measurement of performance and outcome factors is a process itself, subject to variation, errors, and potential improvement. An integrated data system effectively becomes part of the clinical process it measures. Experience has shown that many (as much as 30 to 50 percent for some processes) of the assignable outlier points identified within new processes, when tracked to root causes, arise because of the measurement

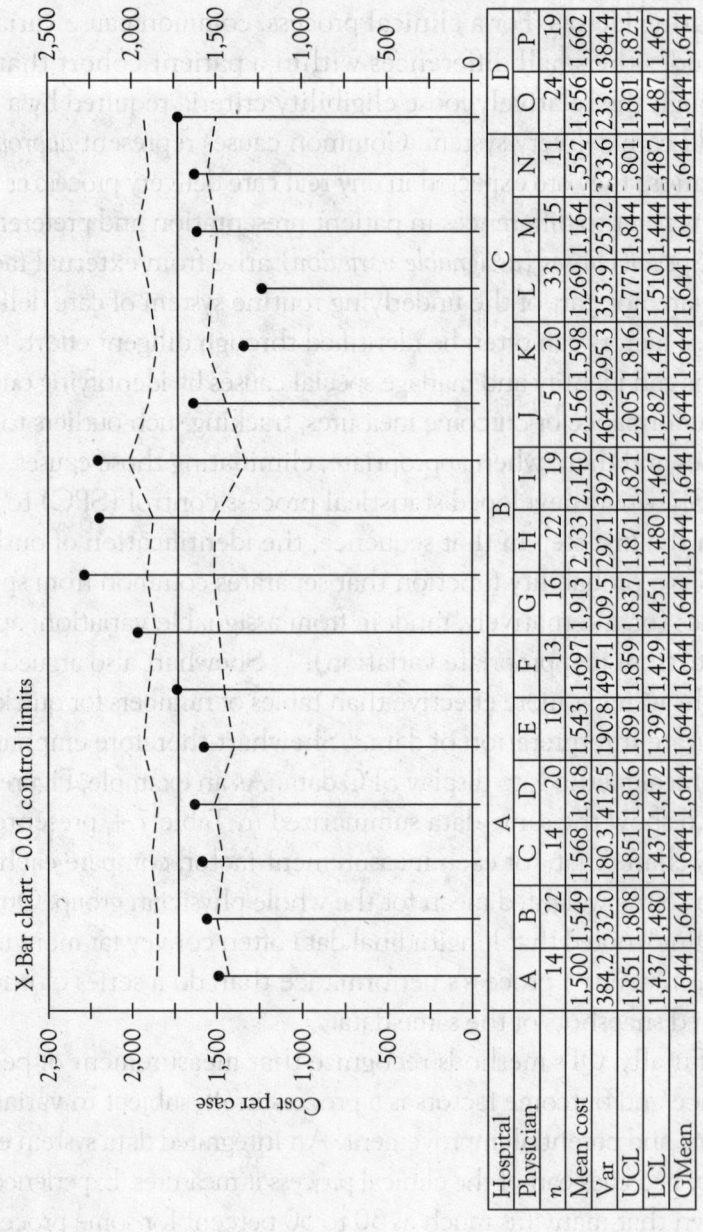

FIGURE 7.2 Total Cost per Case

X-Bar chart - 0.01 control limits

Hospital	A				B					C				D		
Physician	A	B	C	D	E	F	G	H	I	J	K	L	M	N	O	P
n	14	22	14	20	10	13	16	22	19	5	20	33	15	11	24	19
Mean cost	1,500	1,549	1,568	1,618	1,543	1,697	1,913	2,233	2,140	2,156	1,598	1,269	1,164	552	1,556	1,662
Var	384.2	332.0	180.3	412.5	190.8	497.1	209.5	292.1	392.2	464.9	295.3	353.9	253.2	233.6	233.6	384.4
UCL	1,851	1,808	1,851	1,816	1,891	1,859	1,837	1,871	1,821	2,005	1,816	1,777	1,844	801	1,801	1,821
LCL	1,437	1,480	1,437	1,472	1,397	1,429	1,451	1,480	1,467	1,282	1,472	1,510	1,444	487	1,487	1,467
GMean	1,644	1,644	1,644	1,644	1,644	1,644	1,644	1,644	1,644	1,644	1,644	1,644	1,644	1,644	1,644	1,644

Cost per case

S chart - 0.01 control limits

Variance in cost per case

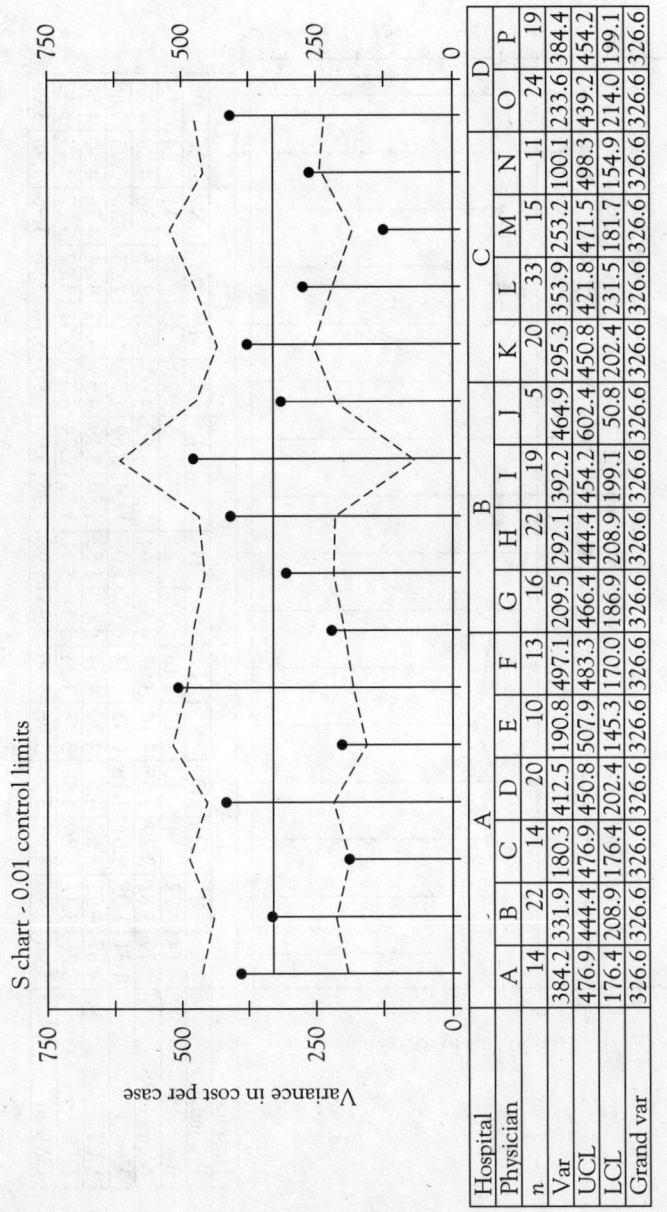

Hospital	A						B				C				D	
Physician	A	B	C	D	E	F	G	H	I	J	K	L	M	N	O	P
n	14	22	14	20	10	13	16	22	19	5	20	33	15	11	24	19
Var	384.2	331.9	180.3	412.5	190.8	497.1	209.5	292.1	392.2	464.9	295.3	353.9	253.2	100.1	233.6	384.4
UCL	476.9	444.4	476.9	450.8	507.9	483.3	466.4	444.4	454.2	602.4	450.8	421.8	471.5	498.3	439.2	454.2
LCL	176.4	208.9	176.4	202.4	145.3	170.0	186.9	208.9	199.1	50.8	202.4	231.5	181.7	154.9	214.0	199.1
Grand var	326.6	326.6	326.6	326.6	326.6	326.6	326.6	326.6	326.6	326.6	326.6	326.6	326.6	326.6	326.6	326.6

FIGURE 7.3 Length of Hospital Stay

X-Bar chart - 0.01 control limits

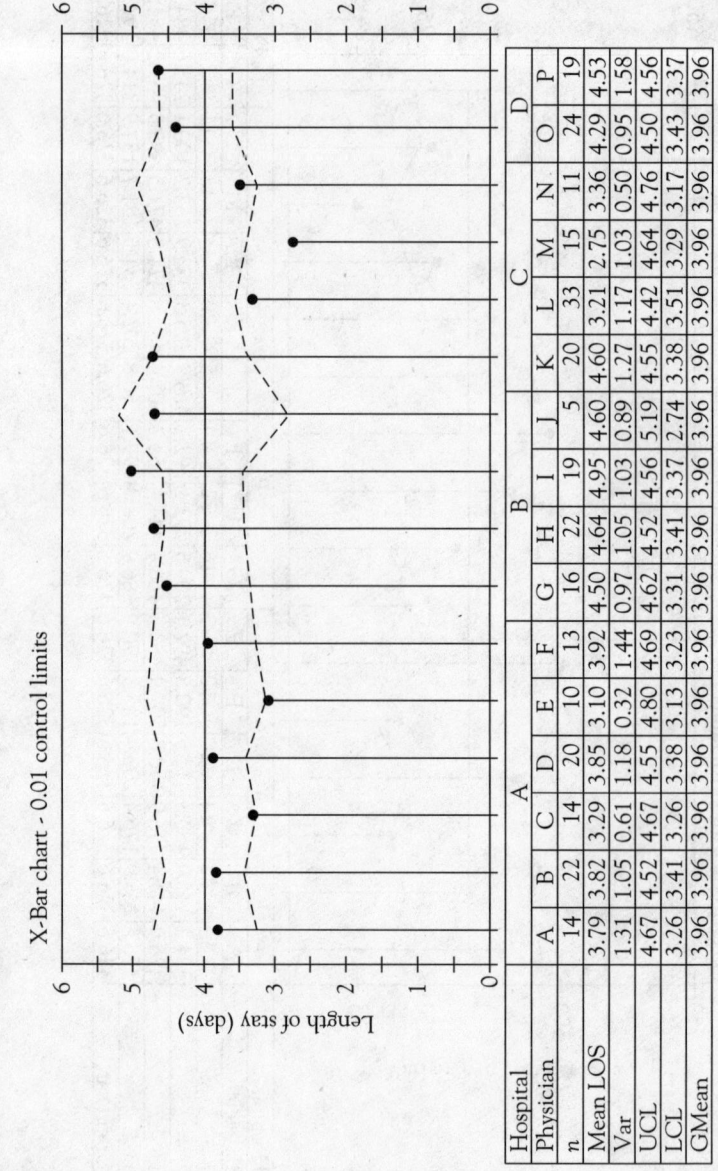

Hospital	A						B					C			D	
Physician	A	B	C	D	E	F	G	H	I	J	K	L	M	N	O	P
n	14	22	14	20	10	13	16	22	19	5	20	33	15	11	24	19
Mean LOS	3.79	3.82	3.29	3.85	3.10	3.92	4.50	4.64	4.95	4.60	4.60	3.21	2.75	3.36	4.29	4.53
Var	1.31	1.05	0.61	1.18	0.32	1.44	0.97	1.05	1.03	0.89	1.27	1.17	1.03	0.50	0.95	1.58
UCL	4.67	4.52	4.67	4.55	4.80	4.69	4.62	4.52	4.56	5.19	4.55	4.42	4.64	4.76	4.50	4.56
LCL	3.26	3.41	3.26	3.38	3.13	3.23	3.31	3.41	3.37	2.74	3.38	3.51	3.29	3.17	3.43	3.37
GMean	3.96	3.96	3.96	3.96	3.96	3.96	3.96	3.96	3.96	3.96	3.96	3.96	3.96	3.96	3.96	3.96

Length of stay (days)

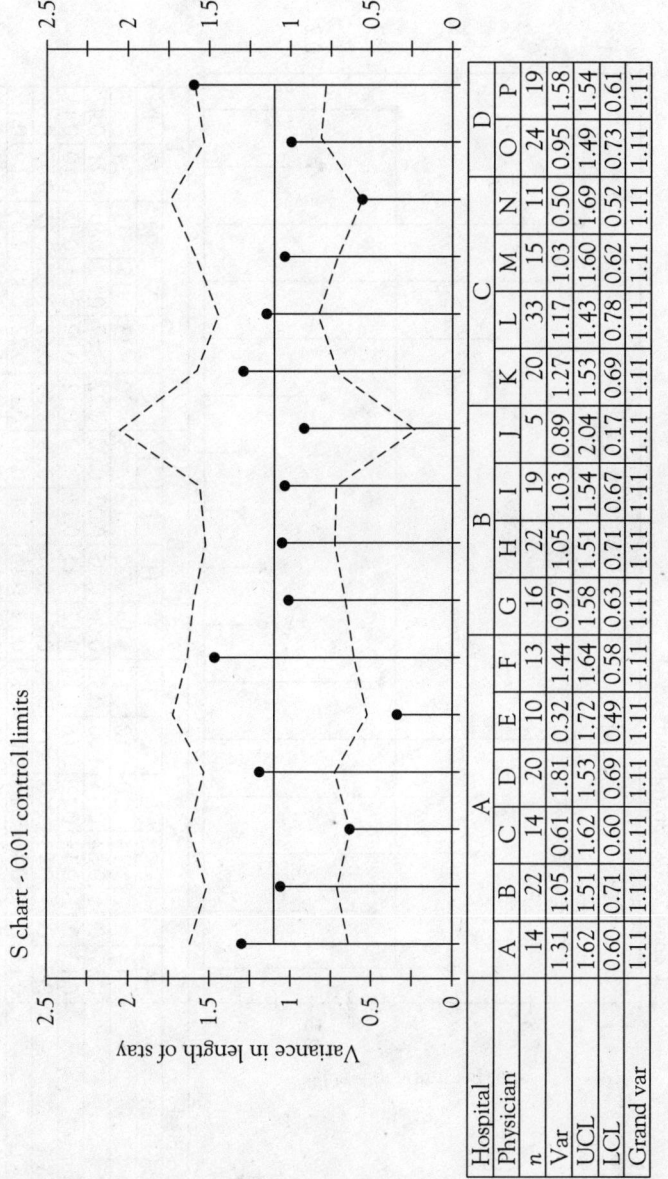

S chart - 0.01 control limits

Variance in length of stay

Hospital	A						B					C				D
Physician	A	B	C	D	E	F	G	H	I	J	K	L	M	N	O	P
n	14	22	14	20	10	13	16	22	19	5	20	33	15	11	24	19
Var	1.31	1.05	0.61	1.81	0.32	1.44	0.97	1.05	1.03	0.89	1.27	1.17	1.03	0.50	0.95	1.58
UCL	1.62	1.51	1.62	1.53	1.72	1.64	1.58	1.51	1.54	2.04	1.53	1.43	1.60	1.69	1.49	1.54
LCL	0.60	0.71	0.60	0.69	0.49	0.58	0.63	0.71	0.67	0.17	0.69	0.78	0.62	0.52	0.73	0.61
Grand var	1.11	1.11	1.11	1.11	1.11	1.11	1.11	1.11	1.11	1.11	1.11	1.11	1.11	1.11	1.11	1.11

FIGURE 7.4 Day of Admission Surgery

P chart - 0.01 control limits

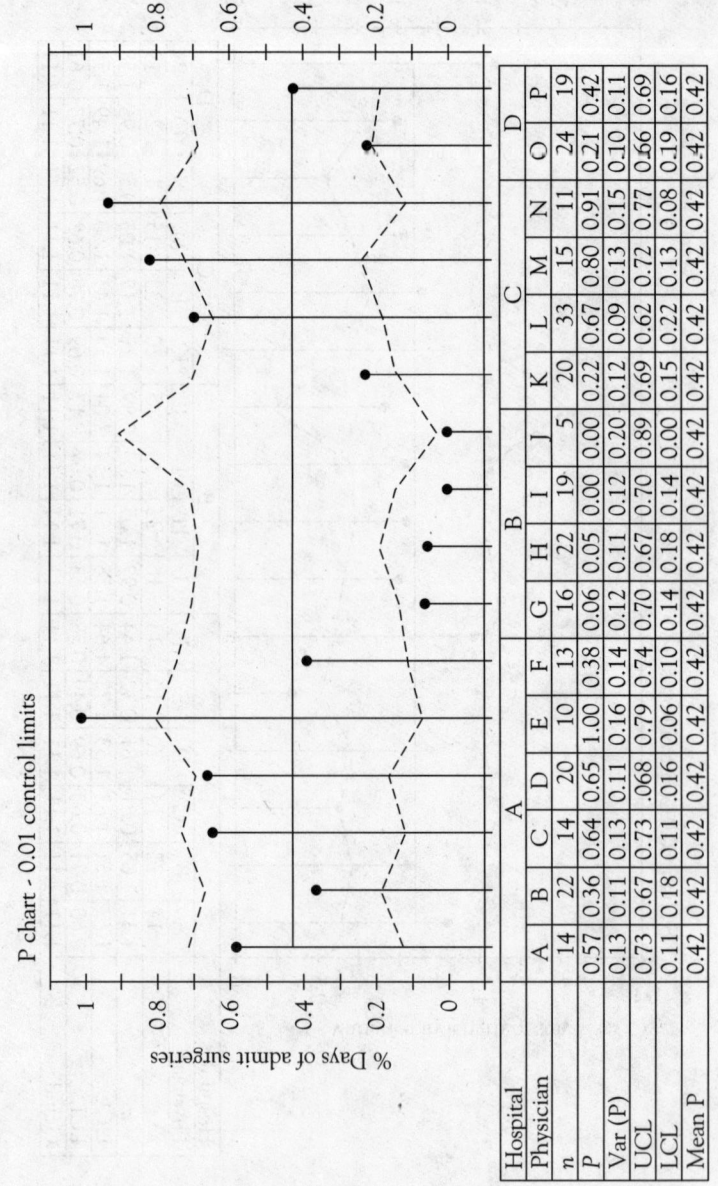

Hospital	A						B				C				D	
Physician	A	B	C	D	E	F	G	H	I	J	K	L	M	N	O	P
n	14	22	14	20	10	13	16	22	19	5	20	33	15	11	24	19
P	0.57	0.36	0.64	0.65	1.00	0.38	0.06	0.05	0.00	0.00	0.22	0.67	0.80	0.91	0.21	0.42
Var (P)	0.13	0.11	0.13	0.11	0.16	0.14	0.12	0.11	0.12	0.20	0.12	0.09	0.13	0.15	0.10	0.11
UCL	0.73	0.67	0.73	.068	0.79	0.74	0.70	0.67	0.70	0.89	0.69	0.62	0.72	0.77	0.66	0.69
LCL	0.11	0.18	0.11	.016	0.06	0.10	0.14	0.18	0.14	0.00	0.15	0.22	0.13	0.08	0.19	0.16
Mean P	0.42	0.42	0.42	0.42	0.42	0.42	0.42	0.42	0.42	0.42	0.42	0.42	0.42	0.42	0.42	0.42

% Days of admit surgeries

FIGURE 7.5 Grams of Prostatic Tissue Excised

X-Bar chart - 0.01 control limits

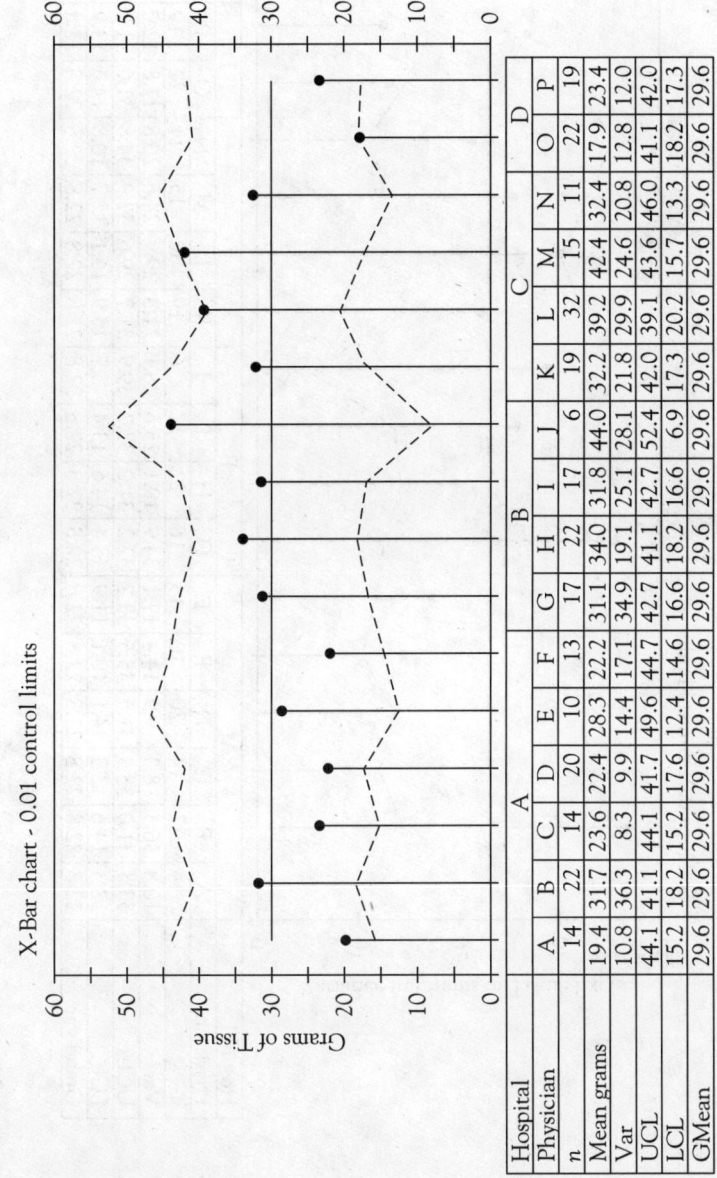

Hospital	A						B				C				D	
Physician	A	B	C	D	E	F	G	H	I	J	K	L	M	N	O	P
n	14	22	14	20	10	13	17	22	17	6	19	32	15	11	22	19
Mean grams	19.4	31.7	23.6	22.4	28.3	22.2	31.1	34.0	31.8	44.0	32.2	39.2	42.4	32.4	17.9	23.4
Var	10.8	36.3	8.3	9.9	14.4	17.1	34.9	19.1	25.1	28.1	21.8	29.9	24.6	20.8	12.8	12.0
UCL	44.1	41.1	44.1	41.7	49.6	44.7	42.7	41.1	42.7	52.4	42.0	39.1	43.6	46.0	41.1	42.0
LCL	15.2	18.2	15.2	17.6	12.4	14.6	16.6	18.2	16.6	6.9	17.3	20.2	15.7	13.3	18.2	17.3
GMean	29.6	29.6	29.6	29.6	29.6	29.6	29.6	29.6	29.6	29.6	29.6	29.6	29.6	29.6	29.6	29.6

Grams of Tissue

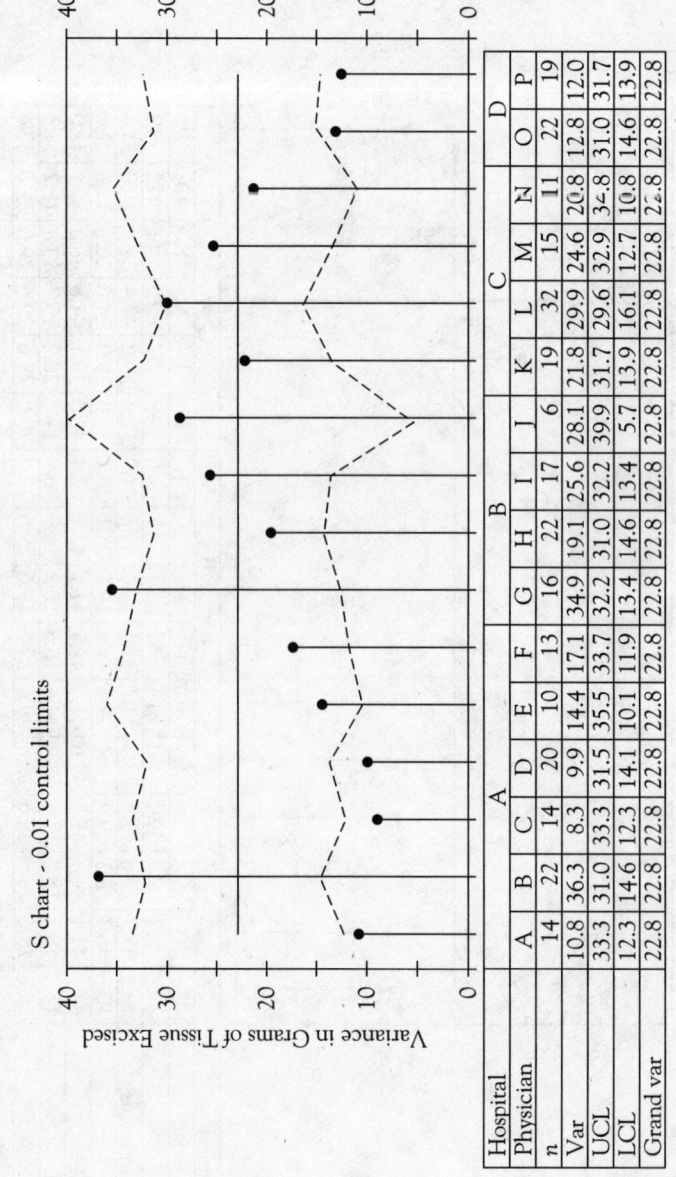

FIGURE 7.5 Grams of Prostatic Tissue Excised, Cont'd.

S chart - 0.01 control limits

Variance in Grams of Tissue Excised

Hospital	A						B					C			D	
Physician	A	B	C	D	E	F	G	H	I	J	K	L	M	N	O	P
n	14	22	14	20	10	13	16	22	17	6	19	32	15	11	22	19
Var	10.8	36.3	8.3	9.9	14.4	17.1	34.9	19.1	25.6	28.1	21.8	29.9	24.6	20.8	12.8	12.0
UCL	33.3	31.0	33.3	31.5	35.5	33.7	32.2	31.0	32.2	39.9	31.7	29.6	32.9	34.8	31.0	31.7
LCL	12.3	14.6	12.3	14.1	10.1	11.9	13.4	14.6	13.4	5.7	13.9	16.1	12.7	10.8	14.6	13.9
Grand var	22.8	22.8	22.8	22.8	22.8	22.8	22.8	22.8	22.8	22.8	22.8	22.8	22.8	22.8	22.8	22.8

FIGURE 7.6 Surgical Procedure Time

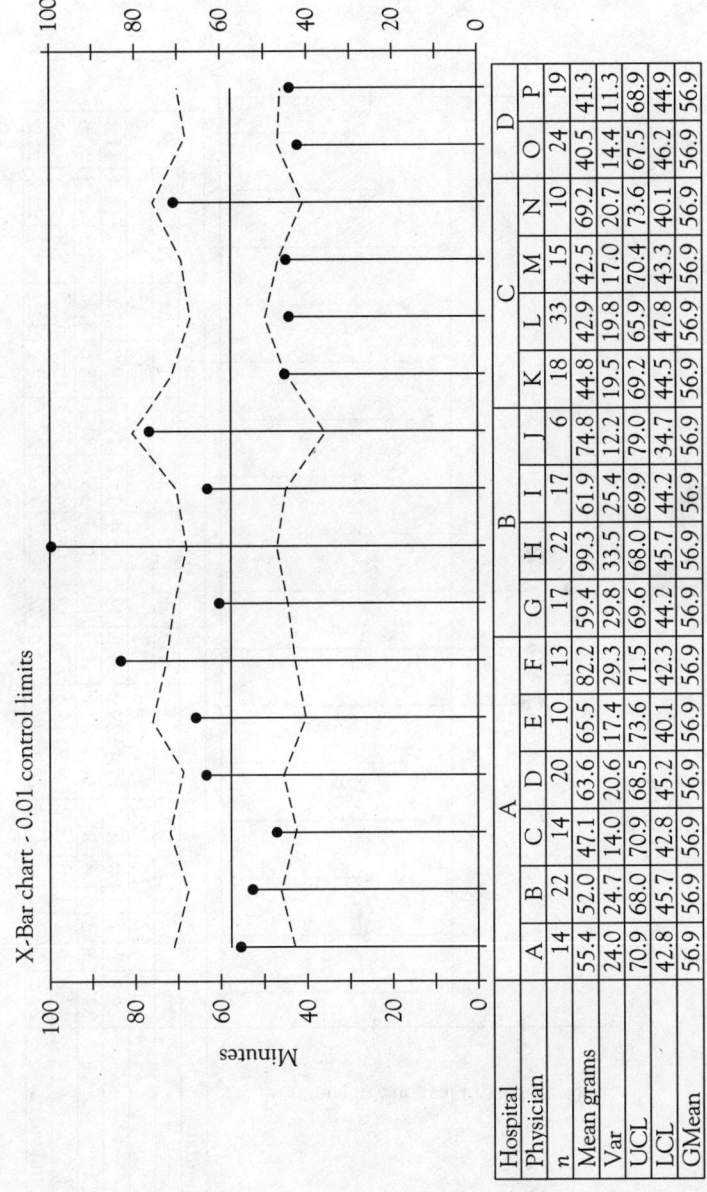

X-Bar chart - 0.01 control limits

Hospital	A						B				C				D	
Physician	A	B	C	D	E	F	G	H	I	J	K	L	M	N	O	P
n	14	22	14	20	10	13	17	22	17	6	18	33	15	10	24	19
Mean grams	55.4	52.0	47.1	63.6	65.5	82.2	59.4	99.3	61.9	74.8	44.8	42.9	42.5	69.2	40.5	41.3
Var	24.0	24.7	14.0	20.6	17.4	29.3	29.8	33.5	25.4	12.2	19.5	19.8	17.0	20.7	14.4	11.3
UCL	70.9	68.0	70.9	68.5	73.6	71.5	69.6	68.0	69.9	79.0	69.2	65.9	70.4	73.6	67.5	68.9
LCL	42.8	45.7	42.8	45.2	40.1	42.3	44.2	45.7	44.2	34.7	44.5	47.8	43.3	40.1	46.2	44.9
GMean	56.9	56.9	56.9	56.9	56.9	56.9	56.9	56.9	56.9	56.9	56.9	56.9	56.9	56.9	56.9	56.9

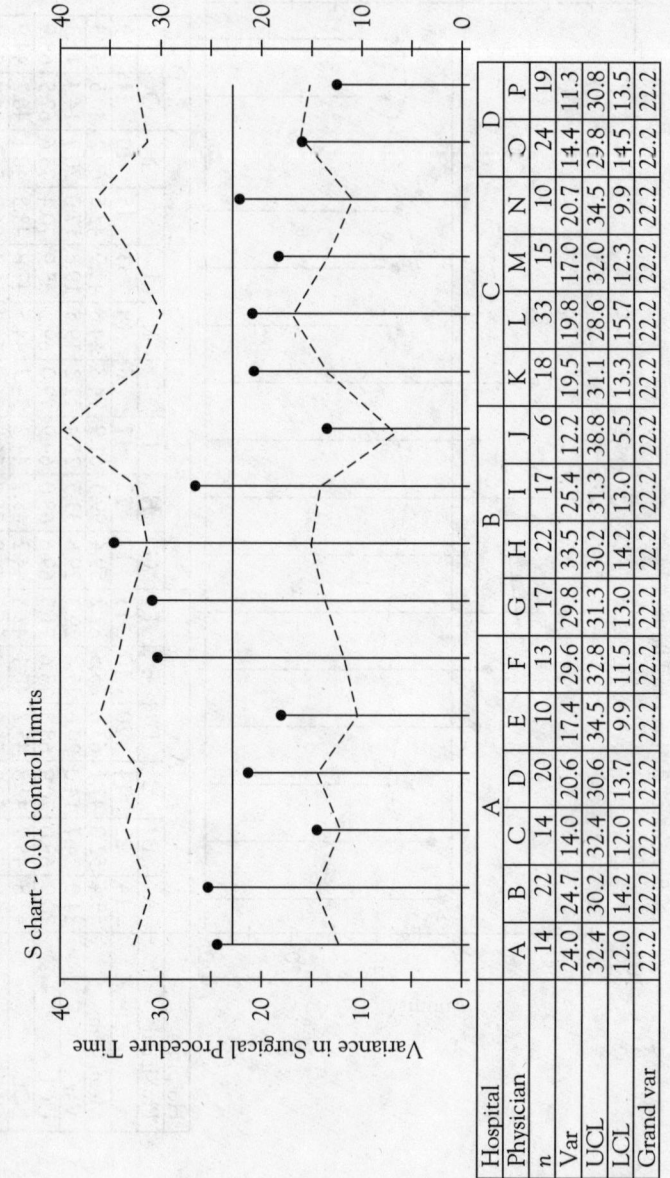

FIGURE 7.6 Surgical Procedure Time, Cont'd.

S chart - 0.01 control limits

Variance in Surgical Procedure Time

Hospital	A					B					C				D	
Physician	A	B	C	D	E	F	G	H	I	J	K	L	M	N	O	P
n	14	22	14	20	10	13	17	22	17	6	18	33	15	10	24	19
Var	24.0	24.7	14.0	20.6	17.4	29.6	29.8	33.5	25.4	12.2	19.5	19.8	17.0	20.7	14.4	11.3
UCL	32.4	30.2	32.4	30.6	34.5	32.8	31.3	30.2	31.3	38.8	31.1	28.6	32.0	34.5	29.8	30.8
LCL	12.0	14.2	12.0	13.7	9.9	11.5	13.0	14.2	13.0	5.5	13.3	15.7	12.3	9.9	14.5	13.5
Grand var	22.2	22.2	22.2	22.2	22.2	22.2	22.2	22.2	22.2	22.2	22.2	22.2	22.2	22.2	22.2	22.2

system itself, rather than stemming from the process of care. Iterative techniques that can stabilize clinical performance over time can simultaneously stabilize the process's measurement system as well.

Conclusions

The TURP study reported in this chapter was actually the first step in a QI study design. The study results were blinded (James[33] presents the theory showing why the data were blinded) and then presented in urology staff meetings at three of the four participating hospitals (the fourth hospital served as a control). A follow-up study conducted nine months later showed significant declines in physician-to-physician variation in length of stay, cost per case, true surgical procedure times, grams of prostatic tissue removed, and many other performance indicators, as compared with a control group, in each of the three hospitals where data were shared. The cost of a TURP fell by about 15 percent in the three institutions. Many other groups now anecdotally report similar experiences when physicians receive, in a nonthreatening setting, valid clinical data regarding their care delivery practices compared with those of their peers. At that level, QI methods may look like case management to a hospital administrator, and they often can earn their way at that level alone.

QI methods, however, go far beyond case management. When properly implemented, they represent an alternative study design that is very closely related to traditional health services research methods. More than that, through ideas like iterative stabilization of process and measurement factors, control of bias factors through direct measurement, graphical methods to feed back performance data to process operators over time, and integration into routine care delivery processes, QI methods make significant contributions to variation analysis and outcomes research. They represent another way of balancing control of bias, generalizability, and practicality and add one more important tool for those who would address Western medicine's immense need for valid information to guide clinical decisions and performance.

Notes

1. Glover, J. A. (1938). The incidence of tonsillectomy in school children. *Proc R Social Medicine, 31*, 1219–1236.

2. Lewis, C. E. (1969). Variations in the incidence of surgery. *New England Journal of Medicine, 281*(16), 880–884.

3. Wennberg, J. E., & Gittelsohn, A. (1973). Small area variations in health care delivery. *Science, 182*, 1102–1108.

4. Wennberg, J. E., Barnes, B. A., & Zubkoff, M. (1982). Professional uncertainty and the problem of supplier-induced demand. *Social Science and Medicine, 16*(7), 811–824.

5. Wennberg, J. E. (1985). Variations in medical practice and hospital costs. *Connecticut Medicine, 49*(7), 444–453.

6. McPherson, K., Wennberg, J. E., Hovind, O. B., & Clifford, P. (1982). Small-area variations in the use of common surgical procedures: An international comparison of New England, England, and Norway. *New England Journal of Medicine, 307*(21), 1310–1314.

7. Chassin, M. R., Kosecoff, J., Park, R. E., Winslow, C. M., Kahn, K. L., Merrick, N. J., Keesey, J., Fink, A., Solomon, D. H., & Brook, R. H. (1987). Does inappropriate use explain geographic variations in the use of health care services? A study of three procedures. *Journal of the American Medical Association, 258*(18), 2533–2537.

8. Park, R. E., Fink, A., Brook, R. H., Chassin, M. R., Kahn, K. L., Merrick, N. J., Kosecoff, J., & Solomon, D. H. (1986). *Physician ratings of appropriate indications for six medical and surgical procedures* (R-3280-CWF/HF/PMT/RWJ). Santa Monica, CA: RAND.

9. Chassin, M. R., Brook, R. H., Park, R. E., Keesey, J., Fink, A., Kosecoff, J., Kahn, K., Merrick, N. J., & Solomon, D. H. (1986). Variations in the use of medical and surgical services by the Medicare population. *New England Journal of Medicine, 314*(5), 285–290.

10. Leape, L. L., Park, R. E., Solomon, D. H., Chassin, M. R., Kosecoff, J., & Brook, R. H. (1990). Does inappropriate use explain small-area variation in the use of health care services? *Journal of the American Medical Association, 263*(5), 669–672.

11. Eddy, D. M. (1992). *A manual for assessing health practices and designing practice policies.* Philadelphia: American College of Physicians.

12. Henke, C. J., & Epstein, W. V. (1991). Practice variation in rheumatologists' encounters with their patients who have rheumatoid arthritis. *Medical Care, 29*(8), 799–812.

13. Sage, W. M., Kessler, R., Sommers, L. S., & Silverman, J. F. (1988). Physician-generated cost-containment in transurethral prostatectomy. *Journal of Urology, 140,* 311–315.

14. Gillespie, K. N., Romeis, J. C., Virgo, K. S., Fletcher, J. W., & Elixhauser, A. (1989). Practice pattern variation between two medical schools. *Medical Care, 27*(5), 537–42.

15. Eagle, K. A., Mulley, A. G., Field, T. S., Skates, S., Bero, G., Clark, C. E., Sexton, J. O., Reder, V. A., Berrigan, G., Procaccini, J., & Thibault, G. E. (1991). Variation in intensive care unit practices in two community hospitals. *Medical Care, 29*(12), 1237–1245.

16. Eddy, D. M. (1984). Variations in physician practice: The role of uncertainty. *Health Affairs, 3,* 74–89.

17. James, B. C. (1993). Implementing practice guidelines through clinical quality improvement. *Frontiers of Health Services Management, 10*(1), 3–37.

18. Angell, M. (1993). Caring for women's health: What is the problem? *New England Journal of Medicine, 329*(4), 271–272.

19. Neuhauser, D. (1991). Parallel providers, ongoing randomization, and continuous improvement. *Medical Care, 29*(Suppl. 7), JS5–JS8.

20. Institute of Medicine. (1990). *Clinical practice guidelines: Directions for a new program.* Washington, DC: National Academy Press.

21. Roos, N. P., Wennberg, J. E., Malenka, D. J., Fisher, E. S., McPherson, K., Andersen, T. F., Cohen, M. M., & Ramsey, E. (1989). Mortality and reoperation after open and transurethral resection of the prostate for benign prostatic hyperplasia. *New England Journal of Medicine, 320*(17), 1120–1124.

22. Sidney, S., Quesenberry, C. P., Sadler, M. C., Cattolica, E. V., Lydick, E. G., & Guess, H. A. (1992). Reoperation and mortality after surgical treatment of benign prostatic hypertrophy in a large prepaid medical care program. *Medical Care, 30*(2), 117–125.

23. Elwood, P. M. (1988). Shattuck Lecture—Outcomes management: A technology of patient experience. *New England Journal of Medicine, 318*(23), 1549–1556.

24. Greenfield, S. (1989). The state of outcomes research: Are we on target? [Editorial]. *New England Journal of Medicine, 320*(17), 1142–1143.

25. Concato, J., Horwitz, R. I., Feinstein, A. R., Elmore, J. G., & Schiff, S. F. (1992). Problems of comorbidity in mortality after prostatectomy. *Journal of the American Medical Association, 267*(8), 1077–1082.

26. Berwick, D. M. (1991). The double edge of knowledge [Editorial]. *Journal of the American Medical Association, 266*(6), 841–842.

27. Shewhart, W. A. (1986). *Economic control of quality of manufactured product*. Washington, DC: Ceepress. (Original work published 1931)

28. Berwick, D. M. (1991). Controlling variation in health care: A consultation from Walter Shewhart. *Medical Care, 29*(12), 1212–1225.

29. James, B. C., Horn, S. D., & Stephenson, R. A. (in press). *Management by fact: The relationship of quality improvement to outcomes management, practice guidelines, and randomized clinical trials*.

30. Ryan, T. P. (1989). *Statistical methods for quality improvement*. New York: Wiley.

31. Ott, E. R., & Shilling, E. G. (1990). *Process quality control: Troubleshooting and interpretation of data*. New York: McGraw-Hill. (Original work published 1975)

32. Cleveland, W. S. (1985). *The elements of graphing data*. Monterey, CA: Wadsworth.

33. James, B. C. (1992). Good enough? Standards and measurement in continuous quality improvement. In *Bridging the gap between theory and practice* (pp. 1–24). Chicago: Hospital Research and Education Trust (American Hospital Association).

PART THREE

Policy and Management

8

Physician Involvement in Quality Improvement

Issues, Challenges, and Recommendations

Stephen M. Shortell, Ph.D.

It is widely believed that the systematic application of industrial quality management science principles and practices can result in marked improvements in the quality, productivity, and outcomes of medical care.[1,2,3] Yet, most of the applications of these principles and practices to date have been in nonclinical areas such as scheduling systems, billing practices, and administrative support services.[4]

Financial support for the National Survey of Hospital Efforts to Improve Quality was provided by the Baxter Foundation, Deerfield, Ill., under a grant to the Center for Health Services and Policy Research at Northwestern University. Appreciation is expressed to Deborah Bohr, Chris Izui, and Peter Kralovec of the Hospital Research and Educational Trust (HRET) and the American Hospital Association Survey Data Center for fielding the questionnaire. Financial support for conducting the case studies was provided by the Center for Health Management Research of the Western Network and the National Science Foundation. Appreciation is expressed to the following ten case study sites for their time and cooperation: Catherine McAuley Health System, Ann Arbor, Mich.; Good Samaritan Hospital, Kearney, Neb.; Good Samaritan Regional Medical Center, Phoenix, Ariz.; LDS Hospital, Salt Lake City, Utah; McKay-Dee Hospital, Ogden, Utah; Providence Medical Center, Portland, Oreg.; St. Clare Hospital, Tacoma, Wash.; St. Vincent Hospital, Portland, Oreg., Tucson Medical Center, Tucson, Ariz.; and Virginia Mason Medical Center, Seattle, Wash. Appreciation also is expressed to the following individuals who assisted the study team in conducing various interviews: David Blumenthal, M.D., M.P.P.; Jennifer Edwards, Dr.P.H., M.H.S.; Frank Lefevre, M.D.; Joel Shalowitz, M.D., M.M.; and Howard Zuckerman, Ph.D. The research assistance of Jeff Erdman and the manuscript preparation assistance of Alice Schaller and Margaret Kaffenberger are gratefully acknowledged.

In fact, some have referred to this application as committing a Type III error—namely, solving the wrong problem.[5] Commonly cited barriers to clinical application of industrial quality management science (also referred to here as "continuous quality improvement"/ "total quality management" [CQI/TQM]) include the inherent complexity of many medical care processes, physicians' relative inexperience in working with teams and in delegating responsibility, and a general lack of physicians' understanding and support. This failure to find clinical applications for CQI/TQM is unfortunate because it is in the application of CQI/TQM to clinical processes that the largest impact can be made.

As part of a larger study of quality improvement in U.S. hospitals, investigators at Northwestern University (Evanston, Ill.), the University of California (Berkeley), and the University of Colorado (Denver) are examining the issue of physician involvement in CQI/TQM through both survey methods and ten in-depth comparative case studies. Among the issues addressed in this chapter are (1) documentation of the degree of physician involvement in CQI/TQM activities, (2) assessment of the kinds of clinical applications currently undertaken, (3) examination of the perceived impact of such activities to date on costs and patient outcomes, (4) analysis of differences according to whether or not the hospital is formally and behaviorally committed to CQI/TQM, and (5) development of an overall framework for assessing hospital quality improvement efforts, including specific recommendations for increasing the degree of effective physician involvement in such efforts. Where appropriate, differences are assessed by bed size, teaching orientation (residency program affiliation), and whether or not the hospital is a member of a system.

The National Survey

The survey, completed by each hospital's CEO and person in charge of quality improvement, was sent to all 5,492 of the nation's nonfederal, nonspecialty care hospitals; 3,303 provided complete useable responses, for a response rate of 60 percent.[6,7,8] Responding hospitals were somewhat larger (220 versus 170 beds), were more likely to be teaching hospitals (8.8 percent versus 4.2 percent), and were somewhat more likely to be members of health care systems (41 percent versus 35 percent) than nonresponding hospitals.

As part of the questionnaire, respondents were asked to indicate whether they had formally incorporated CQI/TQM into their institutions. Positive responses to each of the following items was taken as indicative of formal commitment to CQI/TQM: (1) a philosophy of continuous improvement of quality through improvement of organizational processes, (2) use of *structured* problem-solving processes incorporating statistical methods and measurement to diagnose problems and monitor progress, (3) use of teams including employees from multiple departments and from different organizational levels as the major mechanism for introducing improvement in organizational processes, (4) empowering employees to identify quality problems and improvement opportunities and to take action on these problems and opportunities, and (5) an explicit focus on "customers"—both external and internal. Using these indicators, approximately 69 percent of hospitals reported active involvement in CQI/TQM activities; the majority (73 percent) of these, however, did so only within the past two years.

Physician Involvement

Overall, 43 percent of hospitals reported conducting at least some physician training in CQI/TQM. But, as shown in Table 8.1, only 14 percent of active staff physicians have been exposed to such training to date, and only 10 percent have or currently are participating in a quality improvement project team. As shown, statistically significant differences were found between the CQI and non-CQI hospitals, with the former having somewhat more active physician involvement than the latter. No differences by teaching orientation or by system membership with regard to training were found. Nonteaching hospitals, however, had a somewhat higher percentage of physicians involved in quality improvement teams than teaching hospitals (16.6 percent versus 13.0 percent), and system hospitals had somewhat more physicians involved in quality improvement teams than nonsystem hospitals (11.6 percent versus 8.3 percent).

Clinical Applications

The vast majority of hospitals, over 70 percent, were not yet examining clinical processes or conditions to a significant extent, although 43 percent had developed or were using at least one clinical protocol, guideline, or pathway. A much higher percentage of CQI/TQM hospitals used clinical algorithms, practice protocols/guidelines, or critical pathways (49.5 percent) than non-CQI/TQM hospitals (29.2 percent). Among CQI/TQM hospitals, the use of clinical algorithms varied significantly by bed size, teaching orientation, and system membership. Staff at large hospitals (more than 400 beds) were much more likely than staff at medium-sized (100–399 beds) or small hospitals (fewer than 100 beds) to have developed or used clinical algorithms, practice protocols/guidelines, and critical pathways (68.7 percent versus 52.7 percent and 34.5 percent, respectively). Also, staff at teaching hospitals were more likely to have developed or used clinical algo-

TABLE 8.1 Findings Pertaining to Physician Involvement

	Overall	CQI hospitals	Non-CQI hospitals
Percentage of active staff physicians receiving formal QI training	14.0	16.2*	9.5
Percentage of active staff physicians participating in QI projects	10.0	10.1*	8.4

* $p \leq .05$.

rithms, practice protocols/guidelines, and critical pathways (65.9 percent) than staff at nonteaching hospitals (47.6 percent). Finally, staff at hospitals belonging to systems were more likely to have developed or used protocols and pathways than those not belonging to systems (56.7 percent versus 43.5 percent).

Table 8.2 shows those conditions for which quality of care data are most frequently used by specific quality improvement project teams. These range from approximately 27 percent for pneumonia to nearly 44 percent for coronary artery bypass surgery (CABGs). In all cases, staff at CQI/TQM hospitals were more likely to use quality data in improvement work than staff at non-CQI/TQM hospitals. Examining only CQI/TQM hospitals, no significant differences were found in use of quality data by project teams on the basis of either teaching orientation or system membership. Staff at large hospitals, however, were more likely than staff at medium-sized and small hospitals to use quality of care data for total hip replacements (47.0 percent versus 33.7 percent versus 24.2 percent, respectively). This pattern also was found for angioplasty: staff at 36.6 percent of the large hospitals and at 38.2 percent of the medium-sized hospitals used quality of care data in quality assurance/quality improvement (QA/QI) project teams versus staff at only 22.2 percent of the smaller hospitals.

On average, all hospitals used quality of care data in QA/QI project teams for 17.7 percent of the fifteen listed conditions/procedures performed by the hospital. For CQI/TQM hospitals, this figure was 20.3 percent versus only 11.8 percent for non-CQI/TQM hospitals. Among CQI/TQM hospitals, the percentage of conditions for which quality of care data were used by QA/QI project teams differed significantly by bed size but not by teaching orientation or system membership. Project teams at large hospitals were more likely to use quality of care data (23.7 percent) than at small hospitals (20.5 percent) and medium-sized hospitals (19.3 percent).

Hospital respondents also were asked to indicate whether they used both clinical and cost data in reviewing physician privileges and credentials. Results show that a much higher percentage of

TABLE 8.2 Percentage of Hospitals Reporting Use of Quality of Care Data by Organized QA/QI Project Teams

	All Hospitals	CQI/TQM hospitals	Non-CQI/TQM hospitals
Coronary artery bypass surgery	43.9	46.5*	32.8
Cesarean section	32.5	36.0*	24.0
Total hip replacement	29.9	34.3*	16.4
Angioplasty	28.8	31.2*	18.3
Pneumonia	26.7	31.1*	16.9

$*\ p \leq .05.$

CQI/TQM hospitals used both clinical and cost data in reviewing physician privileges and credentials than non-CQI/TQM hospitals (34.8 percent versus 20.8 percent).

Among CQI/TQM hospitals, the use of clinical and cost data in reviewing privileges and credentials varied by bed size, teaching orientation, and system membership. Specifically, large hospitals (51.9 percent) were more likely to use such data than medium-sized hospitals (36.1 percent), which, in turn, were more likely to use such data than small hospitals (24.1 percent). Teaching hospitals were more likely to use such data than nonteaching hospitals (58.8 percent versus 32.0 percent), and hospitals belonging to systems were more likely to use such data than those not belonging to systems (38.5 percent versus 31.5 percent).

Perceived Impact

Patient and Related Outcomes. Survey respondents were asked to indicate on a scale of one (low) to seven (high) the impact of their hospital's QA and QI activities on a number of items that form three scales: human resource development, patient care outcomes, and financial outcomes. The human resource development scale was calculated by averaging responses to the following items: (a) reduced employee turnover, (b) improved management skills and practices, (c) improved hospital-physician relations, (d) increased physician commitment to the hospital, (e) increased nursing staff satisfaction, (f) greater employee empowerment, (g) increased ability to recruit and retain nurses, and (h) increased ability to recruit and retain physicians. The patient care outcomes scale was formed by averaging responses to the following items: (a) improved patient outcomes, (b) reduced errors and inappropriate treatment, (c) increased patient satisfaction, and (d) improved continuity of patient care. Finally, the financial outcomes scale was created with averaged responses to the following items: (a) reduced costs, (b) improved productivity/efficiency, and (c) increased profitability. Each of these scales exhibited high internal consistency and reliability.

In general, CQI/TQM hospitals reported that their QA/QI activities had a greater impact on human resource development and financial outcomes than non-CQI/TQM hospitals. CQI/TQM hospitals, for example, reported a higher degree of impact on the human resource development items than other hospitals (3.32 versus 3.08, respectively). CQI/TQM hospitals also scored significantly higher on the financial outcomes scale than other hospitals (3.66 versus 3.35). No differences were found between the two groups, however, with regard to the perceived impact on patient care outcomes.

Examining only CQI/TQM hospitals, some differences existed by hospital bed size and system membership. For example, hospitals belonging to systems perceived a greater impact on human resource development (3.37 versus 3.26) and on financial outcomes (3.73 versus 3.57) than freestanding hospitals. Also, small hospitals perceived a greater impact on patient care outcomes than large hospitals (4.64 for < 100 beds versus 4.47 and 4.45 for the large categories). However, large hospitals perceived a greater impact on financial outcomes than small hospitals (3.80 for the > 400 bed category versus 3.58 and 3.70 for the other categories). No differences were found on any of the measures by teaching orientation.

Respondents also were asked to indicate the number of statistically significant, measurable improvements in patient outcomes achieved as a result of their QI efforts. The eight areas examined were (1) reduction in overall mortality adjusted for severity of illness, (2) reduction in condition-specific mortality adjusted for severity of illness, (3) reduction in postoperative wound infection rates, (4) reduction in cesarean section (C-section) rates, (5) reduction in unplanned readmission rates to the ICU, (6) reduction in medication errors, (7) reduction in inappropriate use of blood products, and (8) increase in patient satisfaction survey scores. The results for the most frequently reported items (shown in Table 8.3) suggest that CQI/TQM hospitals were more likely to report increases in patient satisfaction and reductions in C-section rates than non-CQI/TQM hospitals, but no differences were found in reduction of inappropriate use of blood products or reduction in postoperative wound infection rates. Interestingly, non-CQI/TQM hospitals were somewhat more likely to report reduction in medication errors than CQI/TQM hospitals. Overall, CQI/TQM hospitals reported statistically significant improvements for an average of 1.9 of the items listed versus 1.75 for non-CQI/TQM hospitals. Bed size, teaching orientation, and system membership did not have significant effects on the above results.

Cost Savings. Respondents were asked to indicate the number of statistically significant, measurable cost savings achieved as a result of their QI efforts in twelve hospital departments, including admitting, ambulatory surgery, anesthesia, billing, emergency, laboratory (including blood bank), medical records, operating room, outpatient services, patient care units, pharmacy, and radiology and also whether the average length of stay (overall or for a particular condition) was significantly reduced. Table 8.4 indicates five areas in which cost savings were most frequently reported. As indicated, a higher percentage of CQI/TQM hospitals reported cost savings

TABLE 8.3 Percentage of Hospitals Reporting Statistically Significant Improvements in Patient Outcomes

	All Hospitals	CQI/TQM hospitals	Non-CQI/TQM hospitals
Reduction in medication errors	40.4	39.3	42.9
Increase in patient satisfaction scores	38.8	40.4*	35.3
Reduction in inappropriate use of blood products	37.8	37.8	38.0
Reduction in postoperative wound infection rates	27.8	28.0	28.4
Reduction in cesarean section rates	23.4	25.3	19.3

*$p \leq .05$.

in every area than non-CQI/TQM hospitals. Overall, CQI/TQM hospitals reported a significantly higher number of departments in which cost savings had been achieved than non-CQI/TQM hospitals (2.29 versus 1.55). For those experiencing cost savings, the majority reported saving less than $100,000.

Among the CQI/TQM hospitals, system member hospitals were likely to report a higher number of departments with cost savings than nonmembers (2.45 versus 2.11). Also, large hospitals reported more departments with cost savings (2.69) than either medium-sized (2.21) or small hospitals (2.22). This finding is consistent with the earlier observation that large hospitals perceived a greater impact on overall financial outcomes than small hospitals.

Summary of National Survey Data

At present, physician involvement is relatively slight in either QI training or participation in QI project teams, although, as expected, the involvement is somewhat greater among hospitals formally

TABLE 8.4 Percentage of Hospitals Reporting Statistically Significant, Measurable Cost Savings

Department	All Hospitals	CQI/TQM hospitals	Non-CQI/TQM hospitals
Significantly reduced average length of stay	29.6	32.2*	23.8
Pharmacy	24.9	26.8*	20.7
Laboratory (including blood bank)	21.3	23.2*	17.2
Patient care units	19.1	21.8*	12.9
Billing	18.1	20.1*	13.6

* $p \leq .05$.

involved with CQI/TQM than among those not involved. Of special note is the significantly greater involvement of CQI/TQM hospitals in clinical applications involving use of clinical data to improve quality for specific clinical conditions and procedures; use of protocols, guidelines, and pathways; and use of clinical and cost data in reviewing privileges and credentials. Among CQI/TQM hospitals, the large hospitals, teaching hospitals, and hospitals belonging to systems are significantly more likely to be involved in clinical applications than the small hospitals, nonteaching hospitals, and hospitals not belonging to systems.

The above differences in physician involvement and clinical applications between CQI/TQM hospitals may be important because the data also suggest that CQI/TQM hospitals report experiencing a more positive impact on human resource development issues (for example, hospital-physician relationships and physician commitment to the hospital) and financial outcomes than non-CQI/TQM hospitals. Further, CQI/TQM hospitals are generally more likely to report statistically significant improvement in some specific patient outcomes and to report cost savings than hospitals not involved in CQI/TQM activities. These findings suggest that efforts to increase meaningful physician involvement in CQI activities are likely to have a positive impact. Some suggestions for achieving greater physician involvement are examined in the following section.

The Case Studies

As part of a larger study of QI implementation, ten case studies were conducted that included examination of issues related to physician involvement and clinical applications.[9] The ten sites were selected on the basis of variation in experience with formal CQI/TQM efforts and included four hospitals with no formal CQI/TQM experience, four hospitals with one or two years of experience, and two hospitals with more than two years of experience. The same definition of CQI/TQM was used for the case study analysis as was used in the national survey. The hospitals ranged in size from 60 beds to 618 beds, with an average bed size of 383. Occupancy rates ranged from 52 to 82 percent, with an average of 65 percent. Seven sites had residency training programs, and eight were members of systems. Overall, the hospitals were involved in CQI/TQM for an average of 3.6 years.

Methods

The site visits were conducted during a three-day period by a team of three to five members made up of a combination of physicians and social scientists. Interviews were conducted with the chairs of hospital boards; senior administrative leaders, including physicians, quality management leaders, and committee members, typically including several physicians; and QI project team leaders and members, including physicians as appropriate. In addition, data were collected on each hospital's QI plans, reports, results to date, and related information. Among the topics covered were implementation approaches, achievements to date, reasons for success, barriers and obstacles, physician involvement issues, information and analysis issues, empowerment and incentive issues, and future plans.

Physician Involvement Issues: Major Findings

The major findings that emerged from the comparative case studies are highlighted in Table 8.5. Consistent with the national survey results, relatively little physician involvement was found among the case study sites. However, those sites with more experience in formal CQI/TQM efforts had a greater degree of physician involvement than the other sites. Also, the four sites that had focused their QI efforts on *clinical applications* from the beginning had a greater degree of physician involvement, as might be expected, than those that did not. Physician leadership was found to be a key factor influencing physician involvement and acceptance. In addition, physicians were almost universally more comfortable with data-driven clinical studies—particularly with those focused within their own specialty—than with the notion of hospitalwide or organization-wide QI or of developing a continuous improvement culture.

TABLE 8.5 Major Findings of Case Studies Concerning Physician Involvement

- Overall, physician involvement to date is not widespread.
- Somewhat more involvement occurs among hospital-based physicians and procedurally-oriented physicians.
- Physician managers generally are involved and receive early training.
- Physician leadership is key.
- Four sites focused their quality improvement efforts on *clinical applications* from the start; six *did not*.
- Physicians are more comfortable with data-driven clinical studies within their specialty than with the notion of developing an organizationwide, continuous improvement culture.

Among the major reported barriers to physician involvement were the following: (1) physicians were skeptical about hospital motives; for example, many of the case study sites focused their QI efforts—even those in clinical areas—on reducing costs; (2) many physicians did not see the relevance of the hospital's efforts to their own practices; as one interviewee expressed, "It's okay if the hospital wants to do it, but it doesn't affect me"; (3) most physicians reported lack of time as a problem; (4) overall, a lack of relevant clinical data and analysis hindered the ability to address clinical processes and problems of interest to physicians; (5) generally, physician peer group support for involvement was lacking; and (6) some feared that formal QI efforts that resulted in requirements for strict adherence to clinical protocols might be used against them in terms of malpractice threats.

Recommendations

On the basis of the case study interviews and analysis, related observations, and existing literature[10,11,12], a number of recommendations are proposed (see Table 8.6 for a summary). There appears to be considerable debate over how to time the involvement of physicians in CQI/TQM: whether to train them in CQI/TQM early and involve them from the outset or to begin later on in the process after the hospital has gained experience. We believe that a nucleus of physicians should be trained and involved from the beginning to provide an overall sense of physician ownership of the process and to create a nucleus of leaders for further rollout. This group of physicians should include formal physician leaders but, in addition, should include other key clinicians throughout the organization. Typically, this might represent a group of ten to thirty physicians, depending on medical staff or physician group size. The remaining physicians, by far the larger group, would receive just-in-time training consistent with their needs and interests. This training would be conducted by the nucleus of physician leaders noted above. In discussions, it is important to avoid using CQI jargon and, instead, to emphasize clinical practice principles and issues familiar to physicians. In settings where clinical service lines exist and are managed jointly by physicians and managers, it is recommended that these individuals receive *joint* QI training that can be reinforced immediately in the practice setting. Where such naturally occurring working relationships between physicians and managers do not exist, it may make more sense to conduct the initial training in separate groups. In either case, it is important that the training not be exclusively didactic, but rather emphasize experimental approaches focused on real problems facing the physicians and/or managers. For example, several of the study sites required that groups of physicians, nurses, and managers bring a specific clinical problem or issue to the training session. One of these problems then would be the focus of the first quality-improvement project team conducted by the group.

A second major recommendation is that hospitals focus on *strategically important* clinical issues/diagnoses/conditions/procedures. Characteristics of such issues include high-cost/high-volume conditions, conditions for which data are reasonably available, conditions for which improvement opportunities exist, conditions for which reasonable cause-and-effect relationships are understood, and increasingly, primary care conditions in which improvements might result in the greatest long-run payoff. Identifying strategically important clinical issues serves as a high motivator for physicians and indicates the hospital administrators' commitment to addressing core clinical care processes.

A third recommendation is that hospital staff consider developing a "clinical outcome assessment unit" (or equivalent) with sufficient support staff. A number of the sites that were farther along in their physician involvement efforts had such units. These units are used for data collection, analysis, and feedback support for clinically oriented QI teams. They also provide ongoing consultation and benchmarking and may engage in research studies of their own. These units can be organized on a systemwide basis for those

TABLE 8.6 Physician Involvement: Some Recommendations

1. Provide early, targeted training/involvement.
   - Some early training of physician leaders to provide a nucleus for further rollout
   - Some "just-in-time" training as physician needs and interests are identified
   - Avoidance of CQI jargon
   - Some joint training of physicians and managers

2. Focus on strategically important clinical issues/diagnoses/conditions/procedures.
   - High cost, high volume
   - Data availability
   - Improvement opportunities
   - "Cause-and-effect" relationships reasonably well understood
   - Primary care a promising area

3. Develop a clinical outcome assessment unit with sufficient support staff.
   - Data collection, analysis, and feedback
   - Consultation
   - Benchmarking
   - Research

4. Invest in clinical/managerial information systems that are relational and real time.

5. Maximize the value of physician time.
   - As consultants to QI teams
   - As part of guidance teams
   - To frame problems and issues, with execution carried out by other members of the team

6. For hospital-based and salaried physicians, align performance appraisal and compensation with QI participation and accomplishment of objectives.

7. Use a segmentation approach to physician involvement and target each segment with a different strategy.

hospitals belonging to systems; for smaller, freestanding hospitals without the resources to develop their own units, consideration might be given to developing a cooperative strategic alliance for a clinical QI resource center.

Fourth, CQI/TQM requires greater investment than we observed in clinical/managerial information systems that are relational in nature and operate in real time. *Relational* describes the ability to link patients and providers across different delivery settings. *Real time* indicates that the information can be used on a concurrent basis to monitor patient treatment and to take corrective action on the spot. This use involves bedside terminals and office terminals with current patient data on test results and responses to therapy. In particular, clinical data are needed that can provide trends on specific patient conditions over time so that appropriate analyses can be conducted.

Clearly, the availability of time is a major issue limiting physician involvement in QI. However, we found several sites making progress on this issue through a number of mechanisms, including (1) using physicians as consultants to QI teams, (2) using them as a part of "guidance teams"—members who serve in a support function to QI teams in areas of their specialized expertise, and (3) using physicians up front to help frame problems and issues, with execution then carried out by others. Eventually, the goal of the fifth recommendation would be to replace current physician time spent in traditional quality inspection, assurance, and review activities with more relevant QI process work. This change would result in no additional time requirements beyond what physicians now spend on traditional QA activities but would provide a greater yield from physicians' efforts. For example, it might be possible for hospital administrators to eliminate some traditional medical/staff committee assignments and obligations and replace these with potentially more meaningful project teams and task forces focusing on QI.

A sixth recommendation involves hospital-based and salaried physicians. Here, we recommend that *performance appraisal and compensation be aligned* with these physicians' participation in QI efforts and accomplishment of specific QI objectives. For example, the incentive pay or bonus pay of hospital-based radiologists might be determined, in part, on the basis of achievement of specific QI process and outcomes goals for the year. Similarly, pay of salaried primary care physician groups might be determined, in part, on the basis of the results of patient satisfaction surveys and process or outcome improvements in such conditions as treatment of asthma and hypertension.

Finally, we recommend using a *segmentation approach* to physician involvement, in which each physician segment is targeted with a specific strategy likely to increase the probability of successful involvement. Further details regarding the segmentation approach are discussed below.

The above recommendations are likely to be particularly effective where the following conditions exist and/or guidelines are followed:

- A reasonable base of trust exists between physicians and the hospital.

- Projects are selected initially that can produce documentable improvements within 90 to 120 days; what staff at one hospital call "biteable chunks."

- Attention is focused on the underlying causes of problems, and not the symptoms.

- Physicians and other caregivers know the difference the data will make (for purposes of diagnosis and treatment) before the data are collected.

- Mechanisms exist for sharing learning across teams.

- Risk management, utilization management, QA, and QI activities and responsibilities are aligned and linked to each other (for example, at some hospitals, a single office or person is in charge of all).

- Attention is focused on core processes that cut across episodes of illness and the continuum of care.

Segmentation Approach to Physician Involvement. Although it is widely recognized that physicians vary considerably by specialty, stage of practice, practice setting, philosophy of treatment, and related variables, seldom do recommendations take such variation into account. On the basis of our case studies and related information, we believe it is important to segment physicians when considering ways of increasing their involvement in QI efforts. Four groups serve as a useful starting point: (1) salaried hospital-based or group practice-based physicians, (2) selected physicians with special interests in QI, (3) high-admitting physicians of high-cost, high-volume conditions, and (4) what might be termed the "neutral" majority. As shown in Table 8.7, we recommend that salaried hospital-based or group practice–based physicians be involved very early on in the process. Because these physicians have a salaried relationship with the institution, incentives can be created for their involvement, and they are more likely to be interested in contributing, particularly in their own area of expertise. Early involvement of such hospital-based or group practice–based physicians can serve also as a positive, tangible sign to other physicians regarding the hospital administrators' commitment to QI and the practical value to physicians of improving quality in such key areas as radiology, laboratory, anesthesiology, the emergency room, and other areas of "high contact" with the voluntary admitting physician staff.

A second group represents those physicians in almost any organization that have a special interest in QI. These individuals represent a "blessing" to the organization. The organization should capitalize on the interest of these physicians. They should be involved very early in training efforts, and they should be supported. From among them will emerge the physician champions for the organization's QI effort.

A third group to target is comprised of high-admitting physicians of high-cost, high-volume conditions. The challenge here is to target a few of these individuals and to encourage them to receive early training. Again, it helps to avoid CQI jargon and, instead, to stress quality, improving practice using scientific principles, and

TABLE 8.7 Segmentation Approach to Physician Involvement

Salaried hospital-based or group practice–based
- Target early.
- Create incentives.
- Focus on their area of expertise.

Selected physicians with special interests in quality
- Use them; every hospital has a few.
- Support them.

Leading admitters of high-cost, high-volume conditions
- Target a few.
- Avoid CQI jargon.
- Stress quality.
- Emphasize what they believe they need to do to remain competitive.

The "neutral" majority
- Be patient and opportunistic.
- Use physician peer leaders to influence.
- Use fairly short, "just-in-time" training.
- Make sure support systems are in place.

emphasizing what the physicians believe they need to do to remain competitive in their practice. The key is to recognize physicians' positions and to build on their concerns and interests.

Finally, for the vast majority of physicians practicing in hospitals, we use the term *"neutral" majority*. These physicians are usually not against QI efforts, but rather do not see such efforts as relevant to themselves or to their practice. The strategy here is to be patient *and* opportunistic. Wait until these physicians identify problems, issues, or concerns, and then provide them with just-in-time training and exposure to physician peer leaders who already have received QI training. Some hospital administrators have made progress with their physicians by using CQI/TQM principles and practices to streamline office support services such as patient scheduling, billing, and follow-up contacts. For the neutral majority of physicians, it is important that the QI support systems be in place, particularly with regard to the availability of data, necessary statistical consultation and analytical support, and related support mechanisms. Failure to have these support systems in place at this stage will discourage this majority of physicians from ongoing participation and halt whatever progress has been achieved.

Although the above recommendations emerge out of our current research, they are largely supported by case examples of other institutions as well.[11,12] In addition, it is important to note that the rapidly evolving integrated health care systems, with their greater emphasis on managed care and creating value for purchasers, represent a positive sign for greater physician involvement in QI. State and national health reform proposals, of course, add a further incentive. In brief, it should be much easier to involve physicians in systematic QI efforts in the future as the demands for accountability grow and as physicians become more closely associated with integrated delivery systems of one form or another.[13]

Physician Involvement and Organizationwide Quality Improvement

Although this chapter is focused on the challenges posed by physician involvement in CQI/TQM and applications to clinical processes, it is important that these issues be linked to the hospital and health systems' overall efforts to continuously improve quality. Exclusive focus on physician involvement or a few specific clinical conditions only furthers the bifurcation, fragmentation, and suboptimization that currently characterize most health care QI efforts. In fact, exclusive focus on an isolated piece of the overall puzzle might be thought of as committing the Type IV error, mistaking the problem for the solution! Given the growing complexity and interdependence of medical care processes and the trend to provide more care outside the hospital setting, the great need is to involve all caregivers—physicians, nurses, and therapists—and their managerial colleagues in united QI efforts that cut large swaths through the organizational landscape.

Figure 8.1 provides a conceptual framework for addressing organizationwide QI efforts. The "pyramid" of continuous improvement includes cultural, technical, strategic, and structural dimensions. The *cultural* dimension refers to the organization's underlying beliefs, values, norms, and behaviors that can support or serve as barriers to organizationwide improvement. For example, leadership that empowers employees and supports them to act more independently is believed to be a key cultural element of successful QI efforts.

The *technical* dimension refers to the extent to which those associated with the organization have received the necessary training in CQI/TQM tools (for example, cause-and-effect diagrams, process flow diagrams, histograms, statistical process control charts) and group decision-making processes to support QI efforts. The quality of the organization's information systems and data analysis capabilities are also part of the technical component.

The *strategic* component refers to the extent to which the organization's QI efforts are focused on the key strategic priorities of the organization, as opposed to activities that are more peripheral. In other words, to what extent is there a direct link between the organization's QI efforts and what it is fundamentally trying to achieve with its business plan?

FIGURE 8.1 The Pyramid of Continuous Improvement

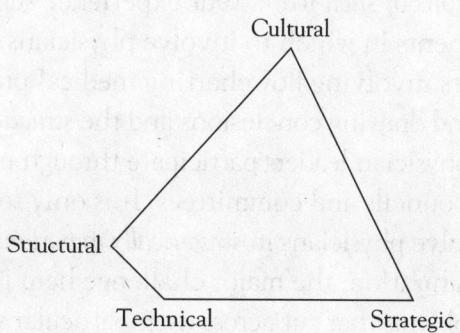

The *structural* element refers to the specific coordinating committees, councils, task forces, and reporting/accountability mechanisms associated with the organization's QI efforts. The structural component brings together the various cultural, technical, and strategic dimensions of the organization's QI work and serves as a forum in which these elements interact.

Primarily on the basis of our experience with the ten comparative case study sites to date, it is our judgment that all four dimensions—cultural, technical, strategic, and structural—need to be addressed in order for significant organizationwide QI to occur. For example, if the cultural component is missing, QI results tend to be short-lived, lacking staying power. Berwick referred to this problem as the "inability to hold the gain."[3] If the technical component is missing, the result may be frustrated efforts on the part of many people who are highly motivated to work on strategically important problems because they are not supported by the necessary tools to be effective. If the strategic component is missing, the result is "pockets of activity" occurring throughout the organization that do not produce any meaningful or significant impact. If the structural component is missing, the organization experiences problems transferring learning throughout the organization and capitalizing on the improvement work that has been done. The four dimensions need to be brought into highly focused alignment with each other for maximum impact to be achieved.

The above discussion suggests that for physicians to be successfully involved in organizationwide QI, they must be *integrated into all four dimensions of such work*. Our experience suggests that the easiest components in which to involve physicians are the *technical* components involving flowcharting medical processes, interpreting data, and drawing conclusions and the *structural components* in which key physician leaders participate through involvement in coordinating councils and committees. It is only somewhat more difficult to involve physicians in *strategically important* clinical issues facing the organization; the major challenge here is getting them to focus on problems that cut across their particular specialty interests. By far the greatest challenge, however, is to involve physicians in the *cultural transformation* believed to be required for organizationwide QI to occur. Physician training and socialization emphasizing individual clinical responsibility and most physicians' traditional independent status from organizations do not provide a foundation for the type of interactive, cross-functional teamwork required of organizationwide QI efforts. But, as population-based capitated health care continues to grow, hospital administrators and physicians increasingly will see their destinies as intertwined, making it easier to bridge their cultural differences. In the meantime, the recommendations previously discussed—using pluralistic segmented training approaches, supporting the emergence of physician champions, providing strong data and analytical support systems, supporting trusting relationships, and so on—can help advance the field in the desired direction.

Notes

1. Laffel, G., & Blumenthal, D. (1989). The case for using industrial quality management science in health care organizations. *Journal of the American Medical Association, 262*, 2869–2873.

2. Berwick, D. M. (1989). Continuous improvement as an ideal in health care. *New England Journal of Medicine, 320*, 53–56.

3. Berwick, D. M., Godfrey, A. B., & Roessner, J. (1990). *Curing health care*. San Francisco: Jossey-Bass.

4. Williamson, J. W. (1991). Medical quality management systems in perspective. In J. Couch (Ed.), *Health care quality management for the 21st century* (pp. 23–72). Tampa, FL: Hillsboro Printing Company.

5. Shukla, R. K. (1994). *Theories and strategies of improving quality and productivity in health care organizations*. Ann Arbor, MI: Health Administration Press, American College of Healthcare Executives.

6. Barsness, Z. I., Shortell, S. M., & Gillies, R. R. (1993, December 5). National Survey of Hospital Quality Improvement Activities. *Hospital and Health Care Networks*, pp. 52–55.

7. Barsness, Z. I., Shortell, S. M., & Gillies, R. R. (1993, December 15). National Survey of Hospital Quality Improvement Activities. *Hospital and Health Care Networks*, pp. 40–42.

8. Barsness, Z. I., Shortell, S. M., & Gillies, R. R. (1994, January 5). National Survey of Hospital Quality Improvement Activities. *Hospital and Health Care Networks*, pp. 45–48.

9. Shortell, S. M., Foster, R. W., Carman, J. M., et al. (1993, June). *New versus traditional approaches to quality improvement: Implementation processes and perceived impact.* Paper presented at the Annual Meeting of the Association for Health Services Research, Washington, DC.

10. Kaluzny, A. D., McLaughlin, C. P., & Kibbe, D. C. (1992). Continuous quality improvement in the clinical setting: Enhancing adoption. *Quality Management in Health Care, 1*, 37–44.

11. McEachern, E. (1993, June). The physician's role in continuous improvement. *The Quality Letter*, pp. 18–21.

12. Gates, P. E. (1993, February). Clinical quality improvement: Getting physicians involved. *Quality Review Bulletin*, pp. 56–61.

13. Shortell, S. M., Gillies, R. R., & Anderson, D. A. (1993, March/April). The holographic organization. *Healthcare Forum Journal*, pp. 20–26.

9

Involving Physicians in Total Quality Management

Results of a Study

David Blumenthal, M.D., M.P.P., and
Jennifer N. Edwards, Dr.P.H., M.H.S.

Despite anecdotal evidence that total quality management (TQM) can improve processes of care and service in large organizations[1,2], many physicians have greeted the tenets of TQM with skepticism.[2,3] Nonetheless, administrators of many U.S. health care organizations are proceeding with efforts to implement TQM on a wide scale. Because of physicians' central role in resource allocation decisions, these administrators will have to develop methods to overcome their physicians' resistance to TQM's philosophy and techniques if they are to succeed. In fact, theory would argue that to realize the full benefits of this new approach to quality management, administrators of health care organizations will have to find ways to make their physicians active, committed supporters of TQM as an approach to improving organizational performance.

In this chapter, we describe results of a qualitative study of how health care organizations with reputations as leaders and innovators

The authors would like to acknowledge the contributions of Ann C. Scheck, who helped conduct several of our case studies. We also wish to express our gratitude for the help we received at each of our participating organizations in planning our site visits and in persuading their colleagues to meet with us. We would like, as well, to thank each of the doctors, nurses, and managers who cooperated so openly and helpfully in the conduct of our work.

in TQM have been responding to the challenge of involving their physicians in TQM. We hope our findings can help health care managers and physician leaders see the applicability of TQM techniques to the work of physicians and, if appropriate, will demonstrate ways to improve the participation of physicians in their organization's efforts to enhance quality and efficiency of care.

Specifically, in this chapter we addresses the following three questions:

1. How involved are physicians in TQM at the current time, and what form has that involvement taken?
2. What factors have facilitated or impeded efforts to involve physicians in TQM and its techniques?
3. What organizational strategies and actions seem to promote or retard the successful recruitment of physicians into TQM activities?

Methods

The observations reported in this chapter are drawn from case studies of six health care organizations that were chosen by using the following criteria:

1. They were varied in type and included hospitals, health maintenance organizations, and multispecialty group practices.
2. They were geographically dispersed.
3. Experts in the field considered them to be advanced and relatively successful in their application of TQM, including their involvement of physicians in TQM activities.

To identify a sample of such organizations, we contacted five experts with national reputations in studying the use of TQM in health care organizations and asked them to list the organizations that met these criteria. Significant overlap among these five lists made selection of the sites fairly straightforward. We invited the staff of two hospitals, two managed care organizations, and two large, multispecialty group practices to participate. The respondent from one group practice declined and consequently that group was replaced with a managed care organization. The organizations selected whose staffs agreed to participate were Intermountain Health Care System, Harvard Community Health Plan, Henry Ford Health System, Group Health Cooperative of Puget Sound, Park Nicollet Health System, and Kaiser Permanente (Ohio Region). A brief description of each is provided in Table 9.1. On visiting these organizations, we discovered that all were evolving into fully integrated health care systems that provided primary, secondary, tertiary, and often home and nursing home care within their communities.

A contact person at each site arranged interviews for us with ten to twenty individuals meeting our designated criteria. The types of personnel we asked to meet with are listed in Table 9.2. The actual people interviewed were selected by our contact person. We and other collaborators visited each site for two or three days in the spring and summer of 1993 to conduct semistructured interviews. Each interview lasted approximately one hour. In most sites, we were allowed to review materials prepared by the organization's staff for their internal use to educate staff about TQM, or materials prepared by staff describing their own TQM projects.

Interviews were recorded, but participants were assured that their comments would not be attributed to them so that they might feel free to critique the strategies pursued by their organization's administrators. Interviews at Intermountain Healthcare were conducted by the two of us in conjunction with a team of researchers led by Stephen Shortell (see Chapter Eight). Interviews at the other five sites were conducted by the two of us plus Ann Scheck, a doctoral candidate in health policy and management, and co-editor of this volume.

Given the overlap of our work with that of Shortell and his

TABLE 9.1 Descriptions of Case Study Sites

1. *Intermountain Healthcare, Inc.—McKay-Dee Hospital*

   This case focused on the Intermountain Health System and one of its member hospitals, the McKay-Dee Hospital. The Intermountain Health System consists of 24 hospitals with 2,800 beds in Utah, Idaho, and Wyoming. McKay-Dee is a 369-bed general medical and surgical hospital located in Ogden, Utah, about 45 miles north of Salt Lake City. McKay-Dee is in the process of building a primary care network as part of its strategy to become a market leader in patient-focused care.

2. *Harvard Community Health Plan*

   HCHP is a mixed staff- and group-model HMO with over 565,000 members and facilities operating throughout Massachusetts and Rhode Island. HCHP operates in one of the most competitive markets in the country. Though it once owned a hospital, it closed that facility in the mid 1980s and now hospitalizes a substantial fraction of its patients at Boston's Brigham and Women's Hospital.

3. *Henry Ford Health System*

   The Henry Ford Health System includes the flagship 903-bed Henry Ford Hospital, an 850-member medical group, an HMO with more than 400,000 members, 32 ambulatory care centers, 3 community hospitals, and a variety of long-term care and home-health-service provider organizations. Since 1983, the system has undergone a number of reorganizations and shifts in relationships between entities. A primary goal of the system's leadership is to integrate these various components while expanding managed care services in southeast Michigan.

4. *Group Health Cooperative of Puget Sound*

   Originally a pure staff-model HMO, GHC now also operates a network-model plan in Eastern Washington and provides almost half its services outside the managed care plan. GHC has 900 physicians and 9,000 employees who provide comprehensive care in 30 primary clinics and several multispecialty centers. A consumer cooperative, GHC has 385,000 participants in western Washington and 90,000 east of the Cascades. The cooperative is heavily influenced by its regionalized structure. Its concerns include competition from other managed care organizations and pressure from purchasers.

TABLE 9.1 Descriptions of Case Study Sites, Cont'd.

5. *Park Nicollet Health System*

Park Nicollet is a mixed health care system that includes a large prepaid health care plan, multispecialty groups that are compensated on a fee-for-service basis, and a 426-bed hospital. PNHS operates 19 outpatient facilities in the Minneapolis–St. Paul area and employs 370 physicians and 2,100 other employees. The system is governed by a 10-member physician board.

6. *Kaiser Permanente—Ohio Region*

Kaiser Permanente is the largest group-model health maintenance organization in the United States. Nationwide, it has more than 6.6 million members. Kaiser Permanente is organized on a decentralized basis, with each region managing its own operations. Management responsibilities are shared by three cooperating entities—the Kaiser Foundation Health Plans, Kaiser Foundation Hospitals, and Permanente Medical Groups.

colleagues, a few comments may be helpful to distinguish the two studies' purposes and methods. Shortell's group undertook a comprehensive study of quality improvement efforts in U.S. hospitals. Their methods involved a survey of all nonfederal hospitals and case studies of ten hospitals that were chosen to include both institutions committed to TQM and institutions with minimal involvement.

Although the study reported in this chapter examined a broader array of health care organizations (HMOs, multispecialty groups, and hospitals) than did that of Shortell and his colleagues, it was more limited in its goals and methods. Our primary purpose was to learn about the involvement of physicians in TQM at organizations known to be leaders in TQM and thereby most likely to illustrate successful strategies for promoting such involvement. Shortell and his coworkers also examined issues pertinent to the involvement of physicians in TQM, though this was not the primary focus of their study. As is evident in this volume, despite very different approaches, the conclusions and observations of the two groups are complementary and similar.

TABLE 9.2 Types of Personnel Interviewed

1. *Senior management*
   Chief executive officer/president
   Chief operating officer
   Chief financial officer
   Chief information officer
   Regional vice presidents
2. *Clinical leadership*
   Medical directors
   Chiefs of services
   Directors of nursing
3. *Quality management staff*
   Director of quality management
   Team facilitators
4. *Physicians, including TQM supporters and others*

Background

Before describing our findings in more detail, it is useful to provide an introduction by explaining how and why the six organizations are pursuing quality improvements through TQM.

How Organizations Have Approached TQM

Berwick (personal communication) has described three ways in which health care organizations become involved in TQM. With reasonable ease, these approaches map on what Shortell and his coworkers describe as the "dimensions of quality improvement." The first approach is *project dominant*, in which managers identify a number of areas for improvement, people are trained in the methods of quality improvement, and teams are created to address particular projects. Teamwork within project groups is emphasized, but no accompanying attempt is made to reorganize the institution as a whole or to revamp its basic culture.

The second approach is *strategy dominant*. Organization managers incorporate quality improvement and meeting the needs of customers into their corporate strategy and business plans. Quality management and a customer orientation become strategic goals and are emphasized and pursued with vigor through a combination of new TQM methods and preexisting managerial tools.

The third approach Berwick describes as *transformational*: senior leadership demonstrates through their own actions that quality is everyone's job and is no longer a separate function of the organization. Training is focused as much—or more—on the philosophy of the organization as on the tools of quality improvement.

In our six sites, we saw elements of each of these approaches to becoming TQM organizations. Some organizations started with one approach and changed to another. Harvard Community Health Plan (HCHP), for example, seems to have moved from an early transformational orientation to a more strategic approach. Intermountain's McKay-Dee Hospital began its quality improvement by organizing project teams, but became strategic, and now seems to be moving toward a transformational approach. Also, within organizations, different subunits and divisions will adopt different methods. As Shortell and his coworkers imply, hybrid approaches may be necessary to foster success in the long run.

Why Now?

Almost all sites had some quality improvement, or at least quality monitoring, system in place prior to the introduction of TQM, but staff at each saw TQM as a departure from the earlier quality management philosophy.

Organizational and environmental factors played critical roles in motivating organizational leaders to adopt a TQM approach to quality management. Staff at all six sites began using TQM between 1988 and 1990. Most sites faced intense competition for patients and needed a way to distinguish themselves from competitors. Kaiser Permanente of Ohio, for instance, had been the low cost option for many employee groups for a number of years and had been able to maintain a sizable market share. The 1980s, however, brought new managed care products into the market, and Kaiser lost its cost advantage. Furthermore, large insurers like Blue Cross/Blue Shield were offering a better rate to group purchasers if they offered the BCBS triple option—the traditional indemnity plan, a PPO, and an HMO—and employers reacted and stopped offering Kaiser to their employees. Management at Kaiser Permanente decided to distinguish their plan from other managed care plans and believed the focus on quality improvement would be a competitive advantage. Senior management interviewed a number of consultants about how to improve quality and found that TQM was a model that fit with their organizational philosophy.

For some, participating in the National Demonstration Project[2] was important to expose leaders to TQM at a time when they were seeking new approaches to enhance organizational performance. Group Health Cooperative faced market pressures similar to those of Kaiser Permanente. A number of senior managers participated in the National Demonstration Project and brought its concepts back to their organization, setting in motion a process that resulted in an organizational commitment to TQM. Others, like Henry Ford Health System, were exposed to TQM through contact with industrial organizations in their immediate environment—in this case, the automobile industry—and saw relevance for their own organizations. Management at Henry Ford recently had acquired many new health care delivery sites and patients and were interested in a corporate strategy that would help them integrate the various provider groups and provide a coherent product focus to present to purchasers and enrollees. For similar reasons, TQM was introduced at Park Nicollet shortly after the merger of the St. Louis Park group practice and the Nicollet group practice and a subsequent management upheaval. TQM was viewed as consistent with the organization's philosophical approach and to have the potential to help Park Nicollet to carve out a niche as a high-quality provider in the Minneapolis–St. Paul market.

None of the organizations we studied adopted TQM simply because it was "the right thing to do" or because it was conceptually or intellectually appealing (though the approach may have had these attractions as well). Administrators at all were seeking to solve particular and pressing organizational needs. Berwick has noted that sometimes a "brush with death" is necessary to motivate staff at a company or health care institution to embark on the radical changes that are required to implement TQM. Executives at none of the organizations we studied had experienced such a drastic threat to survival, but almost all viewed their organizations, then or in the near future, as fighting for positions in an increasingly hostile health care marketplace.

Results

To What Extent and in What Ways Are Physicians Involved in TQM Activities?

All six health care organizations we visited were at the early stages of what their staff believe is likely to be a ten-year (or more) process of becoming TQM organizations. Although all recognize the importance of physician involvement in their organization's evolution toward a TQM culture and in improving clinical care, alternative approaches to promoting this involvement are still being explored, as are the general issues of training, commitment of analytical and financial resources, and organizational strategy development.

Extent of and Approach to Physician Involvement in TQM. Shortell and his coworkers' survey findings that a minority of physicians (10 to 14 percent on average) in their sample institutions had been trained in or had become involved in TQM activities are consistent with the results of our case studies. Low involvement rates seemed to be related as much to management's reluctance to recruit physicians as to physicians' reluctance to participate, though such physician resistance was present as well. In fact, administrators at some institutions were extremely selective and started by approaching only those physicians whom they expected to be receptive.

The one exception to low physician involvement may be HCHP, whose management introduced TQM by attempting to train all of its physicians in the techniques of TQM. As many as 30 to 50 percent of HCHP physicians may have been exposed to formal TQM training. However, HCHP abandoned this approach before staff had completed this comprehensive training effort, in part because of the expense and in part because the organization was not prepared to follow the formal training with specific projects that could involve all trained physicians in quality improvement efforts.

When considering the level of physician involvement in TQM, it should be kept in mind that the organizations studied are very large and that managers at some had adopted the strategy of rolling out TQM in one segment of the organization at a time. In one or two of Henry Ford Health System's Health Centers that were targeted for early exposure to TQM, the majority of physicians had been exposed to TQM by the middle of 1993.

One of the questions that stimulated this study was whether the techniques of TQM were being used by administrators at leading organizations to assist physicians in the management of the clinical problems of individual patients. Blumenthal[4] explored the potential utility of statistical process control, flowcharting, and evolutionary operations in supporting and improving the management of physiological and pathophysiological processes in individual patients. Authors of other chapters in this volume explore applications of TQM techniques in detail (see Chapters Five, Six, and Seven). The reason for emphasizing such approaches to involving physicians in TQM activities is that they may be more appealing to physicians in general, and to physicians-in-training in particular, all of whom are accustomed to thinking about the problems of individual patients. These approaches also may offer opportunities to improve the quality of care by turning data more rapidly and accurately into information that can be used for clinical decision making.

None of the organizations we visited were using TQM in precisely this way. In fact, two-thirds were just beginning to apply TQM to clinical issues, having started by tackling administrative problems. Perhaps the most advanced organizations in addressing clinical issues were the Park Nicollet Health System and Intermountain Health Care; staff at both started their TQM initiatives by trying to improve clinical processes. Administrators at Park Nicollet began their quality improvement initiative by organizing ten clinical quality improvement teams that consisted predominantly of physicians and that were charged with improving the process of care for patients with back pain, chest pain, breast masses, and other presenting problems. Administrators at Intermountain Health Care began tackling clinical issues in the mid-1980s by organizing five RIGHT groups (resource index groups for hospital treatment) that had the goals of reducing costs and improving quality in the management of coronary artery bypass surgery, stroke management, total hip replacement, bowel resection, and cardiac catheterization. Staffed primarily by nurses, administrators, and quality experts, these teams were already in existence when the organization formally adopted TQM as an approach to quality improvement in 1989 and 1990, and the RIGHT groups simply were incorporated into the TQM movement. Consequently, members of the groups received training in TQM techniques and came to view themselves as TQM teams.

In Park Nicollet, McKay-Dee of Intermountain Health Care, and other organizations, clinical improvement initiatives had taken the form of trying to improve systems of clinical care—for example, the process by which breast cancer is diagnosed or the process by which orthopedic patients are postoperatively managed. The logical outcome of such clinical improvement projects is the formulation of guidelines and critical paths for optimal management of classes of patients with particular diagnoses or scheduled for procedures.

Specific Roles of Physicians. Most organizations had recognized three roles for physician participation in TQM: team members, members of a quality council, and opinion leaders.

Team membership. Managers at all sites had organized quality improvement efforts into individual projects to which an interdisciplinary team applied TQM tools. Teams were comprised of health care providers, administrators, and other health care personnel as appropriate to the scope of the problem. Teams had taken varied approaches, but most tried to describe the problem at hand, map (or diagram) the current care process, look for ways to improve it, map a new care process, and implement changes implied by this new care map. In some cases, measuring how the process or outcomes of care changed was the final element.

In all six organizations, doctors participated in both clinical and nonclinical (administrative) quality improvement teams. In the clinical areas, of course, they were indispensable in mapping the current practice, proposing modifications, and implementing changes. For example, physicians provided essential input for a team at Group Health Cooperative that sought to improve the care of diabetes patients. The team initially identified four phases of outpatient care for patients with Type II diabetes and subsequently incorporated eight more aspects of the care process into its care map. This team had access to data to measure the impact of the changed care process on outcomes. Not all teams or organizations have such data available, however, and this is an important problem that managers face when trying to involve physicians in TQM. Results of glycohemoglobin analyses at ten clinics in GHC's South Region were available so that doctors could assess their patients' experiences, compared with others.

When managers of health care organizations used doctors on nonclinical teams, such as appointment scheduling or improving weekend phone access, they did so for two reasons. First, it was an opportunity to train doctors in the methods of TQM and to gain their acceptance. Second, it reinforced the notion of equality of personnel in addressing interdisciplinary problems.

Administrators at Kaiser Permanente Ohio Region used doctors to facilitate all of their teams. They believed that this taught doctors to apply the tools in areas where they do not dominate the discussions and the decisions. The downside of this approach was that it is expensive to have doctors out of their practices for so long (administrators at Kaiser committed four hours per week per doctor for up to two years).

Teams evolved via two routes. Management might identify a number of areas requiring improvement (top-down), or frontline personnel might notice ways to make care processes better (bottom-up). One indicator of the pervasiveness of TQM might be the proportion of teams that are bottom-up. Most clinical and nonclinical teams described to our study team were established or sanctioned by the administration and were supported by facilitators. This apparent tendency toward a top-down approach might reflect a sampling bias because we were interviewing primarily representatives of central administration. In most sites, however, some doctors also were undertaking quality improvement projects on their own. A partial list of areas that study participants described is presented in Table 9.3.

Participation in quality councils. The role of a quality council in a TQM organization is to guide and set priorities in the process of

TABLE 9.3 Examples of Clinical Areas Addressed by TQM Teams at Participating Sites

Affective disorder admissions	Anticoagulation use
Asthma	Back pain
Breast mass evaluation	Cardiac catheterization
Chest pain management	Cholesterol management
Coumadin tracking	Depression
Diabetes	Hypertension
Large and small bowel resection	Mammography protocols
Menopause	Pharyngitis
Smoking cessation	Stroke management
Total hip replacement	Urinary tract infections

implementing TQM, as well as to select teams that will receive the administration's support. Most organizations we visited had either a formal quality council or another managerial body that functioned as its equivalent. The composition of such groups was generally reflective of the management structure and culture. For instance, Park Nicollet is governed by physicians, and physicians dominated the governing board, which had assumed many of the characteristics of a quality council. Kaiser Permanente is a partnership between the Kaiser Health Plan and the Permanente Medical Group. It had a quality council with equal representation of doctors and non-physicians, but the doctors were in the process of creating their own, separate quality group. At both Intermountain and HFHS, hospital management ran the bodies governing decision making about quality projects and invited doctor participation. At Group Health Cooperative of Puget Sound, which has a tradition of lay leadership at the highest levels of the organization, a body called the Delivery System Operating Team provided guidance to quality improvement efforts. This body represented the operational leadership reporting to the chief operating officer of GHC.

Opinion leaders. Doctors who were early converts to TQM played an important role by leading through example: recruiting peers to participate in teams and serving on quality councils. Health care organizations sought out physician leaders for early or supplemental training or to serve on the early TQM teams. Some earned promotions or other leadership positions, in part because of their TQM involvement.

We tried to identify commonly held traits of physician TQM leaders but could not find many similarities across sites. A few had math or engineering backgrounds (both undergraduate and graduate). Hypotheses about younger doctors being most receptive were difficult to test in this type of sample. In some instances, physicians in the middle years of their careers became interested in TQM as a route to change professional direction. Physicians who were employed by health care organizations seemed to accept TQM more readily and were more likely to lead its implementation than were those physicians who worked in affiliated private practices and who had a heightened sense of autonomy. At McKay-Dee Hospital, for example, the physicians working full-time in the intensive care unit assumed leadership roles in quality improvement teams faster than other physicians, though exceptions occurred here as well.

Examples of Physician Involvement in Clinical Problem Solving. At the time of our study, staff at health care organizations across the country were more often applying TQM techniques to nonmedical processes than to clinical processes. A quick review of the literature shows that TQM tools and techniques have been very effective in areas such as streamlining pharmacy work, improving the accuracy of prescription drug distribution to patients, and increasing the speed with which medical records move through health care organizations.

This focus on administrative rather than clinical projects was also characteristic of most of the organizations we visited. Nevertheless, in our case study sites, clinicians told us of dramatic examples of improvements in the processes of patient care. The volume of clinical improvement teams seemed to be proportional to the length of time TQM had been used and the breadth of physician training, an issue discussed later in this chapter. Well-documented and proven successes, however, were relatively rare. Indeed, a consistent problem we encountered was that clinical quality improvement teams have difficulty providing convincing evidence of improvements in quality of care.

When teams measured changes resulting from TQM projects, evidence was generally of two types. First, teams often used patient satisfaction as their primary outcome measure. For staff at most organizations, patient satisfaction was a convenient outcome measure because they already had resources dedicated to patient satisfaction surveys. As a result, they sometimes had baseline data as well.

Second, teams seeking to improve technical quality often measured their effects in terms of process changes. When possible, they also measured decreases in length of stays, use of inappropriate services, and costs or billed charges. Very few were able to measure decreased morbidity or mortality, complication rates, or other clinical outcome measures. Some, however, got close to this goal. The hip replacement team at HFHS showed a shorter time to ambulation as a result of changes in the process of care and the use of a different type of prosthesis. The breast mass team at Park Nicollet reduced the time to definitive diagnosis for new breast masses. These two cases are described below as examples. We also detail the experiences of one of the pediatric asthma teams at HCHP. This team had not produced any measurable results at the time of our study but was notable because it had a high degree of physician involvement.

THE HIP AND KNEE REPLACEMENT TEAM AT HENRY FORD

The hip and knee replacement team at Henry Ford Hospital began as one surgeon's desire to match what he saw as best practice at another hospital. He convened a group of physicians, nurses, social workers, discharge planners, and health plan administrators who were involved in the care of joint replacement patients to look at ways to improve the processes of care. The team had the dual goals to improve care by standardizing methods and to improve satisfaction of those people working with joint replacement patients. Lacking any formal TQM training, the groups took about four months to begin to work together effectively as a team. However, within one year, they had redesigned the care process and had begun treating one surgeon's patients under the new protocol. After a few months of tracking these patients, all three surgeons adopted the same care plan. The revised approach emphasized standardizing preoperative tests and increasing patient education about their expected recovery program. Postoperative care by trained nurses has been increased as well.

After the intervention, inpatient days decreased from a range of seven to ten days per stay to five days. Once home, patients now worked with home health nurses to chart their mobility progress and faxed this information to the surgeon. As a result of the intervention, joint replacement patients were more satisfied with their care. At the time of the study, no adverse outcomes had been documented, and problems were being recognized on a more timely basis.

The team was in the process of assessing the financial impact of shifting patients from inpatient to home care. Some participants in this team were now beginning to investigate ways to improve the functioning of the operating room.

PARK NICOLLET'S IMPROVEMENTS IN EVALUATING BREAST MASSES

The quality council at Park Nicollet selected breast mass evaluation as one of the ten clinical quality improvement initiatives they implemented very early in their TQM activities. A team of nine individuals defined two goals: (1) to reduce variation in evaluating breast conditions so as improve the accuracy, timeliness, and cost of care and (2) to improve the evaluation process to identify breast cancer at its earliest stage. Team members represented gynecology, radiology, surgery, internal medicine, family practice, nursing, and administration. The medical director of the Park Nicollet Clinic served as facilitator during twice-monthly meetings of one and a half hours.

To find the problems in the current treatment for breast masses, the team mapped the care process to identify trouble spots and surveyed patients about their satisfaction with the process. They used formal TQM methods, relying heavily on the FOCUS PDCA (Plan, Do, Check, Act) cycle and on flowcharting both the existing and new processes. Necessary data were abstracted from clinical records. A detailed account of the project was published in the bulletin of the Park Nicollet Medical Foundation.

Through changes in the process of care, the team was able to refer patients more quickly and to reduce delays in diagnosis that caused patients "sleepless nights." The greatest gains resulted from buying and using a Mammotest machine, which enabled radiologists, relying on three-dimensional stereotactic imaging techniques, to place a needle and do a breast mass biopsy in a single session. They adopted the new technique after submitting one hundred women to both old and new diagnostic approaches and finding no difference in detection rates between the two. The team leader reported to us that this new technology probably would have been purchased without the TQM team involvement but that practitioners would not have adopted it as readily because there would have been more rivalry between radiologists and surgeons over which specialty should be responsible for the diagnostic process. In this situation, surgeons permitted radiologists to perform biopsies by using the Mammotest machine.

As a result of changes recommended and implemented by the team, the time period from first evaluation to definitive diagnosis had been reduced from several weeks to two or three days. The total cost savings, if any, had not been calculated, but the cost of the Mammotest procedure was about one-third the cost of a hospital-based biopsy. In addition, 96 percent of breast cancer cases were detected in Stage One of the disease, considered a good clinical result, though the team did not have baseline data with which to compare this new rate.

PLANNING TO IMPROVE THE CARE OF PEDIATRIC ASTHMA AT HARVARD COMMUNITY HEALTH PLAN

As part of a strategic plan to improve quality of care, managers of HCHP assembled a pediatric advisory group to examine pediatric care in the Health Centers Division, the division responsible for its staff model HMO. The pediatric team identified asthma care as an area needing attention because of the high rates of emergency room visits and hospitalization among asthma patients. An asthma team was formed that identified a particular goal: to redesign the medical records of pediatric asthmatics to support chronic and acute asthma management in a way consistent with newly released national asthma guidelines. Using the revised record, all pediatricians would be prompted to reduce variation in management in all settings, encourage interprovider communication, coordinate patient and family education with other aspects of asthma management, and provide clinicians the opportunity to monitor the patients' functional status in a standardized way.

The team members included five pediatricians, an allergist, three physician managers, a director of information services, an analyst, and a nonclinician facilitator. They began by breaking the original project into manageable subproblems. The team followed a formal TQM approach: identifying problems with the current system, brainstorming solutions, defining and surveying its customers, and identifying process improvements.

The team began its work in January 1992 and met regularly until the time when they proposed changes to the electronic medical record (about nine months). As a result, they won the Schering Laboratories Tribute to Excellence Award for their work in developing a process to improve asthma care. They had expected to begin piloting the new medical records system by the summer of 1993, but at the time of our study, the necessary changes in the computerized medical record had not been implemented, so there were no results to report. Meanwhile, the group had moved on to address other asthma concerns, including guideline distribution, baseline measurement, and the design of clinician and patient education programs.

Influences on Extent and Nature of Physician Involvement

We identified eight factors associated with the degree of physician involvement in TQM activities. Undoubtedly, however, there were additional factors we were not able to detect in a sample of this size.

Perceived Relevance of TQM to the Care of Patients. Physicians in our case study organizations held a range of opinions about the relevance of TQM to their work. Many doctors we spoke with (albeit a biased sample) saw the relevance of TQM to their primary concern—patient care—and thought the principles of TQM were consistent with their scientific training. Some noted their appreciation that TQM promotes data-based decision making, empirical experimentation to evaluate proposed changes in process of care, and continuous improvement, rather than a search for a right or wrong approach. A few doctors observed that the methods of TQM could be applied to individual patients and to clinical issues, but others thought TQM was not relevant to the care of individual patients and stated their perception that "it can only be applied to systems."

Doctors who criticized TQM defended the "art of medicine" and the appropriateness of clinical variation. Although fewer physicians than expected attacked the religious zeal with which proponents approached TQM, there is no question that substantial numbers, even in these leading organizations, still lack any exposure to or understanding of TQM, see it as a foreign set of principles, and tend to view adherents as "converts" to a quasi-religious managerial cult. A number expressed the view—explicitly or implicitly—that TQM was simply the latest management fad and would soon pass.

In general, we found that relatively few physicians, aside from a handful of opinion leaders and physician managers, had thought carefully and deeply about the relationship between the techniques of TQM and the process of patient care or had developed a terminology for talking about it with physicians. Many supporters of applying TQM had come to the conclusion that the language of modern quality management should be jettisoned in favor of a pragmatic, data-based approach to solving particular clinical problems one at a time. According to this theory, the jargon of quality management has put off many physicians and obscured its scientific underpinnings. A data-based, problem-specific, and practical approach to solving quality problems is consistent with the way physicians are taught to practice medicine and may very well prove the optimal way to proceed. However, it makes the recruitment of physicians to a "transformational" strategy for implementing TQM extremely difficult. Instead, it tends to institutionalize a project-based approach, thereby limiting the ability of these organizations to accomplish cultural change.

Perceived Leadership. In the industrial setting, leading TQM theorists and practitioners have observed that commitment from senior leadership is vital to the success of TQM efforts. We looked for evidence of such commitment in the organizations we examined, reasoning that it would be essential to overcome the almost inevitable setbacks and problems encountered when attempting to involve physicians in TQM. Given the methods we used to select our study sites, it should come as no surprise that we observed a high level of leadership commitment to TQM. Even in those organizations that recently had experienced a change of leadership, TQM was still being promoted. Senior managers were familiar with the terms and methods of TQM and seemed to understand that they had to play an activist role in quality management in order to accomplish their institutional goals for quality improvement. Many leaders expressed the view that TQM was consistent with good medical practice and did not require a major shift in values or organizational goals. Leaders of these organizations, for the most part, believed that TQM had empowered members of their organizations to question old practices, to innovate, and to listen more carefully to patients and other customers. These attitudinal changes were perceived to be powerful benefits.

Although often fiercely independent, physicians in the organizations we visited were also very sensitive to the messages communicated by leadership with regard to TQM. Several doctors noted that TQM initiatives signaled to them the strong commitment of leadership to quality and that this dedication made them feel supported by the administration to a higher degree than they had been in the past at that institution or in other organizations.

Even in these leading organizations, however, top managers were rarely unanimous or uniform in their embrace of TQM and its principles. At virtually every site, we were told of one or more senior leaders who were "not convinced" but willing to "go along." Not infrequently, these were chief financial officers. In some cases, chief executive officers were described by subordinates as supportive of a general quality thrust but not fully familiar with the content and methods of TQM. In other cases, CEOs were seen as the prime movers, whereas more junior executives were described as skeptics. Some decentralized institutions had managers of major operating units who were openly hostile to TQM, whereas their corporate leaders expressed unequivocal endorsement. In fact, achieving a united front among organizational leaders seemed more difficult in decentralized organizations because of the often enormous variability in the commitment of local leadership to TQM.

Divisions among leaders in their attitudes toward or support of TQM undoubtedly are recognized by physician staff and can contribute to physician passivity or outright resistance. Physicians often lack an appreciation for the complexity of managing a large organization. Particularly discouraging for participants is the failure of leadership to implement recommendations of quality improvement groups or the perceived failure of leadership to commit what physicians perceive to be adequate resources to support the problem-solving teams that have been commissioned by the organization.

Culture. Like their nonphysician counterparts, physicians participate in and are influenced by the traditions, operating style, and values of the organizations in which they work. Doctors at each organization explicitly cited aspects of its institutional culture that improved or hindered the spread of TQM. In one site (HCHP), doctors said they already were accustomed to solving problems in committees and thus found it quite consistent and comfortable to participate in TQM groups. Another site (Kaiser) had a history of separateness between the physicians and all other staff that made it difficult for teams to operate without blaming individuals and minimizing the importance of nonphysicians' contributions. At Intermountain Health Care, a health system that started as a group of Mormon hospitals, the importance of religious values was said to make it easier for the entire organization to make an explicit commitment to quality as a primary organizational goal. At Henry Ford Health System, a tradition of competition among decentralized units tended to make those units more protective of their independence and less likely to embrace central leadership's decision to implement TQM.

Availability of Data and Analytical Support.   Although physicians are not always rigorous or self-critical in their approaches to managing individual patients, they are trained in the scientific method, and they are taught to demand evidence of efficacy before adopting new clinical modalities. Thus, they approach proposed changes in patient management with skepticism and frequently insist on proof that what they currently are doing is inadequate and that proposed alternatives are better.

As a practical matter, overcoming this skepticism and meeting such standards of evidence require the availability of valid data on the performance of existing and revised processes of care. Not surprisingly, therefore, physicians and nonphysicians at all six sites we visited thought that data about processes and outcomes of care were an important element in gaining the support of physicians for TQM teamwork. Such data served several purposes. First, they motivated physicians to participate in quality improvement efforts by identifying clinical situations in which outcomes were suboptimal or where physicians varied greatly in the processes or outcomes of their care for similar patients. As several nonphysician quality management staff confessed, they had virtually no hope of gaining the commitment of physicians to tackle a clinical issue if they could not present valid and convincing evidence that a problem existed. Second, physicians required evidence of improvement in clinically significant parameters before they regarded a TQM project as successful. This was particularly true for skeptics.

A common theme through all of our case studies was that the capacity of the organization to support TQM teams with data and analytical resources was often the rate-limiting step in TQM team progress. Even in the most advanced organizations, users expressed frustration over the limited information and the lack of personnel able to respond to their quality improvement needs.

Organizational leaders were aware of the importance of data collection to TQM activities, in general, and to physician support, in particular. Of the six organizations we visited, two had made major investments in information systems, and two were initiating such efforts. In some organizations, improved information systems will include clinical work stations to support data collection and improved patient management. Perhaps because of these resource commitments, some leaders thought that concerns over the lack of information to document quality problems and to test proposed solutions were overblown and reflected naivete on the part of physicians and other personnel involved in TQM activities. A common comment was, "There will never be enough data to meet everyone's needs."

Creating and managing data systems are expensive activities, and needs often outrun expectations. Nevertheless, we also encountered situations in which the resources allocated to analytical and information support functions seemed disproportionately low in comparison with the ambitious goals and expectations of the organization's TQM programs. In some, the implicit assumption was that teams themselves would collect the necessary data and conduct any required analyses. In fact, many team members accepted this responsibility, performing chart reviews and distributing surveys on their own time, learning how to create histograms and spreadsheets on their own PCs, drawing their own storyboards, and so on. However, this effort resulted in two undesirable side effects. We encountered one senior manager in an organization with a very active TQM effort who confessed that she was spending about a third of her time in front of a computer, manipulating data for her quality improvement team. We also encountered teams that stalled because they were required to wait months for crucial data on existing or reformed processes.

The use of professional and senior managerial personnel as data analysts and the unavoidable delays resulting from insufficient data collection and analysis capabilities affect all personnel involved in TQM. These factors are especially problematical when physicians are team members. As noted below, physicians' time is expensive, and to use them for data collection and analysis or to require them to attend unproductive meetings that are stalled for lack of data may seriously affect organizational efficiency. Furthermore, the tenuous commitment of physicians to quality management can be jeopardized by disappointment and frustration over the slow TQM team progress.

Time. Despite the advantages of involving physicians in TQM, achieving this entails large costs that administrators in many organizations had to weigh. Taking physicians and others away from their regular tasks to work on TQM teams conflicts with most organizations' short-term need to become more efficient. We were told that physicians who did not have a long-term perspective or who were not convinced that leadership was seriously committed to TQM were disturbed about the time they or their colleagues spent on teams. Even when the goals of TQM were widely accepted and supported, systems of care were strained when others had to fill in for TQM team members. In some organizations, physicians participating in TQM activities were required to see more patients in less time or to do their TQM work on the side. Doctors who might have decided to practice in an organized setting because of its controllable hours were struggling with the conflict between their commitment to improve quality and their desire to preserve personal time. At this point, most doctors were cutting into their personal time to participate on teams, but it was recognized that this might not be a sustainable approach.

Administrators at several organizations were pursuing solutions such as hiring staff to fill in and paying departments for their losses. In no cases were doctors experiencing decreases in income because of their team participation. Managers at several organizations talked about reducing doctors' time on teams by using them as consultants, rather than as full team members, and these groups acknowledged trade-offs between team morale and effectiveness. Staff at some organizations were working with compensation schemes designed to alleviate the burden on a physician's colleagues during his or her absence for TQM team activities.

Training. Strategies for training physicians to participate in TQM had not yet been fully developed at the organizations we visited. Our study sites displayed variation in the type, amount, and timing of physician training, and changes of direction were common. Executives at most sites acknowledged that the development of teaching philosophies, methods, tools, and case materials were major challenges that had to be met if they were to be successful in reaching physicians in their organizations.

For some administrators, teaching physicians about the philosophy and tools of TQM had been an important first step. They described three advantages to doing so early on in their TQM implementation. First, embarking on widespread training of physicians (and others) is expensive, thus demonstrating the leaders' commitment to improving quality of care. Second, by training physicians, the administrators are making a symbolic statement that they anticipate that physicians will participate wholeheartedly in improving quality of care. Third, it enables physicians to participate more fully in TQM teams. Nevertheless, at the time of our study, instructors at most organizations had trained only a small group of physician leaders in the philosophy and tools of TQM.

Often, the methods were not explicitly identified as TQM, but instead were embedded in a broader discussion of improving clinical care. Through participation in early teams, the first group of physician trainees was expected to become facile with the techniques and then to teach them to peers. In most cases, trained facilitators were available to assist physicians in applying TQM, though some had the same amount of training as the physicians. Together, the facilitators and the physician leaders provided just-in-time training to other participants.

Administrators at many sites began their training activities by hiring TQM consultants to provide training services. Over time, at three of the sites, those training activities were incorporated within the organization and were tailored more specifically to the organization's culture. The typical model for physician training was a one- or two-day seminar away from the office. About a quarter of this time was devoted to an overview of TQM philosophy; the rest was used to introduce and teach the tools of TQM, such as flowcharts, process control charts, methods to compare processes and outcomes, and system redesign.

Executives at some organizations believed strongly in just-in-time training, providing people participating in TQM work with training in the context of that work. Such an approach was believed to be culturally appropriate and consistent with proven approaches to adult education. Alternatively, executives at some organizations were experimenting with diverse strategies to involve physicians in quality management. They were combining techniques drawn from the literature on how to influence physician behavior, including use of continuing medical education, academic detailing, promotion of opinion leaders, practice guidelines, and feedback from mentors and supervisors.

Most doctors thought they could have used more training, and instructors at some organizations were responding. Several (such as Intermountain, Park Nicollet, and HCHP) were planning a second level of physician training and hands-on experience designed to have a more clinical focus.

Pace of Change/Roll-Out Strategy.   Implementation strategies to involve physicians in TQM were varied. Staff at some organizations had tried a controlled dissemination approach using physician opinion leaders and careful timing of TQM projects. Staff at others had taken the "spray and pray" approach for broadly disseminating the tools and incentives for quality improvement in hopes that the concept and activities would catch on. At each organization, the strategy selected was believed to fit best with organizational culture and management style. However, untrained physicians may be more likely than those with some exposure to TQM to resent their peers' taking time away from work to participate in teams. Organization instructors who train large numbers of physicians early on or who encourage widespread experimentation may experience less physician resistance than those who rely largely on a gradual and selective training process.

A related strategic issue for many organizations had been the choice between using clinical and nonclinical teams at the outset. Organizations that had the greatest success involving physicians seemed to be those that had embraced clinical issues from the beginning. Executives at HCHP used many clinical teams and were able to identify numerous improvements in patient care. Intermountain started with high-volume, high-cost, diagnostic-related groups (DRGs) that proved a difficult initial strategy, but in the process produced measurable improvements that may have improved both physician and management commitment to TQM. Overall, however, we saw little evidence that success in dealing with administrative or managerial problems translated into physician acceptance of TQM.

Project Selection.   A tension exists between choosing projects through a centralized versus a decentralized approach. Because of the sensitivity of involving physicians in TQM, and because of the importance of clinical issues to the organizations, sites we visited had tended to choose clinical projects with more centralized direction. For example, administrators at Park Nicollet, Group Health Cooperative of Puget Sound, and McKay-Dee/Intermountain had chosen clinical projects centrally and then recruited physician and other staff involvement. Their strategy was to pick projects that involved high-cost and high-volume types of care so that improvements were easier to measure and the organizational impact was widespread.

Staff at the McKay-Dee Hospital of the Intermountain chain started with the eight most expensive DRGs and created groups to evaluate and redesign care processes. Their coronary bypass and total hip replacement teams had been relatively successful. Staff at Group Health Cooperative had identified four diagnoses for systemwide quality improvement and had created an entirely new department to support these teams. This initiative was just starting when we visited the organization.

Such top-down projects have an advantage because they tend to be better supported by organizational resources and therefore experience fewer delays. Nevertheless, as the asthma example from HCHP illustrates, even formally mandated teams were not immune to debilitating delays in implementation.

Top officials at all organizations must seek a balance between central control and local initiative, particularly when physicians are involved. In organizations that have emphasized fostering a TQM culture or where TQM ideas have spread more broadly, doctors are encouraged to pursue their own agendas, and problem-solving teams tend to form spontaneously throughout the organization. Local managers become advocates of such efforts. In this bottom-up TQM culture, however, the danger is that an unresponsive central leadership can seriously and negatively affect the commitment of midlevel managers and physicians to quality improvement when needs for organizational time and resources are not met.

Discussion

On the basis of the experiences of six institutions with reputations as market leaders in involving physicians in TQM, we found that health care organizations are still in the early stages of gaining physician acceptance for applying TQM methods and approaches to clinical and nonclinical problems. In retrospect, this finding should come as no surprise. Implementing TQM is an enormously challenging task for any organization, and the requirement to enlist physicians in TQM programs makes an already tough job even more difficult. The reasons are several.

First, the need to recruit physicians to TQM efforts adds to the already considerable up-front costs of implementing a TQM program. The most obvious source of added expense for administrators who wish to involve physicians is related to meeting very high standards of quality in the data collection efforts. Physicians, with their dose of statistical training and inbred skepticism, will often detect and challenge data of uncertain validity. Similarly, staff who are unable to respond intelligently and confidently to such challenges—and particularly, staff who rely on jargon where reasoned discourse is required—will quickly lose credibility among physicians. The practical implications of these potential problems and behaviors are that administrators wishing to initiate clinical quality improvement projects must invest heavily in information systems, highly trained support staff (including physicians interested in managing TQM efforts), and labor-intensive data collection projects, such as surveys and chart reviews.

The resulting expenses contribute to internal organizational tensions in a time of fiscal constraint. Consequently, a natural response is to dole out resources for clinical quality improvement efforts in small, measured doses, awaiting positive results before additional investment; the alternative—massive investment in staff and data—seems burdensome, risky, and likely to shortchange other apparently critical investments in new facilities and systems. Administrators also seek shortcuts, relying on teams to gather their own data and relying on physicians to perform TQM work during their own personal time.

Second, physicians are culturally and organizationally separate from and resistant to traditional management structures and approaches. In this, they may resemble somewhat the scientific and engineering personnel of large, research-intensive industries, such as electronics, chemical and pharmaceutical companies. Physicians expect and are granted a measure of self-governance in most health care organizations. They prize their autonomy and see it as crucial to meeting professional obligations to patients, obligations that are believed to transcend obligations to the welfare of the organizations in which they work. In the extreme case, they are not even employed by the supporting institutions (the situation at McKay-Dee, for example), but merely use the facilities of such organizations for the benefit of their patients. However, even when they are employed by health care organizations and thus do not enjoy economic independence, the physicians' access to a unique body of knowledge, knowledge that is essential to the effective functioning of the organization, confers a measure of autonomy. In many ways, in fact, the physicians' claim to independence within health care organizations rests on the same foundation as their claim to autonomy in the larger society: their status as professionals.[5]

The result of physicians' special status is that lay managers often lack direct control over the incentives and work conditions that affect physician behavior. In addition, they frequently rely on physicians to manage other professionals. Even given unlimited resources to recruit physicians into TQM activities, this lack of control would be a handicap for lay managers. Perhaps even more important, in many ways the special status of physicians in health care organizations may necessitate the development of new technologies and approaches to disseminate the philosophy and tools of TQM. Techniques and precedents refined in industrial organizations may not apply. It is unlikely that Shewhart, Deming, Juran, or their disciples ever anticipated the unique challenges that would be posed by the need to bring the message of quality management science to medical professionals.

The difficulty of recruiting physicians into TQM activities is only further compounded by physicians' general resistance to change[6] and by their fears that the emphasis in industrial quality management sciences on reducing variation in the process of care will compromise both their ability to vary care to meet the needs of particular patients and their ability to innovate.[7] Furthermore, early applications of TQM have been championed by administrators and have been used primarily to address problems perceived as the responsibility of the organization's administration.[2] This use may create problems for dissemination of TQM, however, because physicians are frequently distrustful of administrators and their motivations in health care organizations.[6]

Requirements and Strategies for Involving Physicians in TQM

The art and science of recruiting physicians to participate in TQM activities is still evolving. On the basis of our case studies and other materials, we offer the following recommendations, knowing full well that they may need modification on both general and specific levels in the light of information gained from organizational experiences and because each specific organization faces unique problems and opportunities within the rapidly changing health care environment (marketplace).

1. Be Certain of the Commitment of Senior Leadership to TQM. Even under the best of circumstances, organizational leaders trying to implement TQM strategies will encounter setbacks and problems that will challenge their commitment to their quality improvement approach. In addition, the requirement to recruit physicians to TQM activities increases the attendant costs and risks of implementing TQM. All of the organizations we visited had experienced failures in their TQM projects, both clinical and nonclinical. Teams had stalled and disbanded, parts of the organizations were overtly or covertly resistant, and firm evidence of success was difficult to develop because of the absence of baseline data.

Such difficulties will stress the importance of unified leadership in pursuing a TQM philosophy and also may provide ample excuse to abandon this approach. In most of the organizations we visited, the leadership commitment seemed sufficient to withstand such set-

backs, but it was very clear that, in the absence of such commitment, the process of implementing TQM enjoyed little hope for
success. In the seminars he offered prior to his death, W. Edwards
Deming expressed the view that he personally saw little value in
trying to assist organizations with their TQM activities unless their
leadership had "constancy of purpose." We believe that such leadership commitment will, in fact, prove predictive both of success in
health care organizations in general and of successful clinical application of TQM in particular.

One critical but often overlooked facet of such leadership commitment is support from health care organizations' boards of
trustees. In the face of competition for talented managers and the
pressures of our health care system, turnover among senior executives in health care organizations is considerable. Boards of trustees
provide a critical source of continuity and direction under such circumstances. When judging the organizational commitment to quality improvement, physicians and other personnel will look for
constancy of purpose not only from their chief executive officers
but also from boards of trustees.

2. *Data, Data, and More Data.* Efforts to involve physicians in
TQM activities are likely to be aborted unless implementers can
provide sound evidence that processes of care need improvement
and that attempted changes have been successful. Ultimately, computerized information systems will prove invaluable in providing
the necessary data, but such systems are likely to take years to perfect, even in farsighted organizations (such as Intermountain Health
Care) that already have made sizable investments. Furthermore,
routinely collected data on clinical processes, no matter how
detailed, are unlikely to provide all of the information necessary to
diagnose and treat the multitude of problems—many unantici-
pated—that must be addressed to improve processes of care. Therefore, administrators at TQM organizations must make considerable
up-front investments in ad hoc data collection mechanisms, relying initially on chart review, patient and provider surveys, studies

by industrial engineers, and whatever other methods are necessary and available. Attempts to implement such data collection efforts frequently encounter skepticism from senior managers who want evidence of the success of TQM before they provide the necessary resources. This attitude, however, is likely to delay or doom efforts to recruit physicians into quality improvement activities and institutional efforts to improve the quality of clinical services.

3. Free Physicians to Participate in Teams. Organization executives who are serious about addressing clinical quality improvement must find sustainable and meaningful ways to support physician participation in TQM efforts. An ideal approach to achieving this goal remains to be discovered. However, if administrators pursue the traditional strategy of placing physicians on teams to address clinical problems, they must provide support to the physicians who serve on the teams. Such assistance must include support for their colleagues who are left to handle the increases in their clinical loads that result when TQM participants are absent. Furthermore, physicians should not suffer any decrement in income or quality of life as a result of participating in TQM activities.

4. Avoid the Jargon and Terminology of TQM. With few exceptions, physicians are repelled by the soaring rhetoric and visionary exhortations of true believers in TQM. At least initially, leaders at the organizations we visited experienced more success in recruiting physicians if they emphasized the scientific methods that form the core of TQM's approach to solving quality problems. Tackling practical clinical problems by using data and the experimental method is a comfortable approach for physicians; talk of cultural transformation is not. Also ineffective in gaining physicians' attention are stirring examples of success of TQM in industries outside health care. Correctly or incorrectly, physicians believe that health care problems are fundamentally different from problems encountered by other industrial organizations.

As noted previously, the preferred down-to-earth approach begs the question of how to involve physicians in the more profound changes in organizational culture that TQM ultimately seeks. Methods for making this transition must be developed later, however, after physicians are more comfortable with modern methods of quality improvement.

5. Be Eclectic. We were impressed during our case studies at the attempts of some organizational leaders to move beyond the classical methods of TQM—for example, application of the PDCA cycle and reliance on multidisciplinary problem-solving teams—to draw on all available methods for changing physician behavior to improve quality of care. As noted above, the technologies developed for disseminating TQM within industrial organizations may not be optimal or sufficient for recruiting physicians. However, organizational leaders should not ignore, for example, the increasing amount of medical literature[8] that documents the success of such techniques as reliance on opinion leaders and academic detailing as methods for educating physicians.

6. Do Not Wait to Take on Clinical Issues. Leaders at several of the organizations we visited decided not to apply TQM methods to clinical issues during the initial stages of their TQM activities. The rationale for this approach seems to be that physicians will feel less threatened by modern quality management methods and be less likely to resist them if those methods are used first to tackle administrative issues. Physicians also may be more likely to accept the application of TQM to clinical problems if they have watched it achieve success with improvements in nonclinical areas.

We did not, however, see any evidence that delay in applying TQM to clinical issues brought the organizations any particular advantage. Nor did we encounter any evidence that tackling clinical issues from the outset handicapped the organizations. If anything, the opposite seemed true. The experiences of Intermountain

Health Care and Park Nicollet Health System addressing clinical issues seemed to increase the skill and confidence of their staffs when responding to growing environmental pressures to tackle clinical quality problems. When a group of purchasers in Minnesota sought bids from health care organizations to cover their health care business, Park Nicollet's track record approaching clinical issues gave it an advantage over the competition.

7. *Train More Rather Than Fewer Doctors.* Debate over whether to train most physicians in TQM methods at the outset or to provide only just-in-time training for participants in quality teams is likely to continue for some time. On balance, however, we thought that those organizations in which many physicians had been trained accrued certain advantages as their administrators tried to recruit physicians into TQM activities. For one thing, by exposing large numbers of physicians to modern quality management methods, organizational leaders were likely to identify physicians with a natural sympathy for TQM and its approach early in the process. These physicians could be recruited to serve as team members and facilitators at a time when such support would otherwise be scarce. In addition, when most physicians were trained, even those who were not sympathetic at least understood what their colleagues were doing when they excused themselves from clinical responsibilities to participate in quality improvement efforts.

In the process of training physicians, it is also essential to help them understand and sort through the multiplicity of quality management strategies and techniques that currently are circulating in the health care world. Instructors in some training programs concentrate narrowly on conveying the philosophy and methods of TQM, usually drawing on the methods of Deming, Juran, or one of the other TQM schools. Useful as such training can be, however, it often leaves physicians wondering how the tools of modern quality management relate to the numerous technologies that are touted by policymakers and health services researchers.[9] Such technologies include outcomes research, clinical epidemiology, practice guidelines, medical effectiveness studies, appropriateness studies, and critical pathways. In fact, all of these tools are consistent with and have parallels to the techniques applied by TQM. Unless the similarities and differences between TQM and the use of a particular technology are clarified, however, physicians may confuse TQM with the application of one or a few of these alternative methods. In the case of Park Nicollet, for example, we sensed that some physicians had come to see TQM as synonymous with a series of guideline development projects that the organization was pursuing in cooperation with other provider organizations. As a result, this blurring of boundaries may frustrate long-term efforts to involve physicians in more broad-based quality improvement projects.

8. Engage the Professionalism of Physicians. The special status of physicians as professionals in health care organizations constitutes one of the most important potential obstacles to implementing TQM but also creates one of the most important potential advantages. Physicians highly prize the advantages of professional status and the autonomy it confers, and they are increasingly aware that it is threatened by external political and environment forces. Although their initial responses to such threats may be negative and defensive—and may include resisting the quality improvement thrust of modern health care organizations—thoughtful members of the physician community ultimately will be driven to adopt more positive strategies permitting them to preserve their autonomy. One such strategy is to lead the effort to improve quality, rather than to oppose it: in effect, to preserve old values by applying new methods.[4]

The professionalism of physicians is a potential asset for TQM proponents in yet another way. Most physicians are committed above all to the welfare of their patients. They recognize that such commitment is both a moral obligation and the foundation of their professional legitimacy. If TQM and its methods can be shown to improve patient care through convincing, valid evidence, then physicians will be unable to resist it for long and instead will become its fiercest advocates. In such circumstances, organizational leaders will have more trouble containing the enthusiasm of their physician staffs than in obtaining their commitment to apply modern quality methods.

Notes

1. Kleefield, S., Churchill, W. W., & Laffel, G. (1991). Quality improvement in a hospital pharmacy department. *Quality Review Bulletin, 17,* 138–143.

2. Berwick, D., Godfrey, A. B., & Roessner, J. (1990). *Curing health care: New strategies for quality improvement.* San Francisco: Jossey-Bass.

3. Berwick, D. M. (1989). Continuous improvement as an ideal in health care. *New England Journal of Medicine, 320,* 53–56.

4. Blumenthal, D. (1993). Total quality management and physicians' clinical decisions. *Journal of the American Medical Association, 269*(21), 2775–2778.

5. Starr, P. (1982). *Social transformation of American medicine.* New York: Basic Books.

6. Eisenberg, J. M. (1986). *Doctors' decisions and the costs of medical care.* Ann Arbor, MI: Health Administration Press.

7. Berwick, D. M. (1991). Controlling variation in healthcare: A consultation from Walter Shewhart. *Medical Care, 29*(12), 1212–1225.

8. Soumerai, S. B., McLaughlin, T. J., & Avorn, J. (1989). Improving drug prescribing in primary care: A critical analysis of the experimental literature. *Milbank Quarterly, 67*(2), 268–317.

9. Palmer, R. H., & Adams, M.M.E. (1993). Quality improvement/quality assurance: A framework in putting research to work in quality improvement and quality assurance. *AHCPR* (93–0034).

10

Policy Challenges in Promoting Quality Improvement

John R. Ball, M.D., J.D., and
David Blumenthal, M.D., M.P.P.

In this chapter, we review some of the policy challenges facing members of the medical profession, and quality managers in particular, as they try to encourage a commitment to continuous quality improvement (CQI). In addition, we address the elements necessary for change in physicians' behavior with regard to total quality management (TQM). Physicians seem to have the view that, as a group, they are Jeffersonians: give them all the information, and they will make the right choices. Giving physicians the information needed to improve quality, however, may not be enough. Managers and policymakers need to spend much more time on creating the conditions that will lead to changes in physician behavior. This expenditure of time will require policy interventions that will make information available in a timely way and that will make using that information safer and easier than it is today.

To illustrate our point, we present a series of short stories about frustration with quality assurance and quality improvement. Then, we describe efforts to promote CQI in the American College of Physicians (ACP)—not from the perspective of a membership organization or as a producer of information, but as a business organization. Although there is much discussion of physician skepticism toward quality improvement in clinical settings, this same physician resistance to quality improvement exists in nonclinical areas–with respect, for example, to organizational and business issues.

Policy Issues

The policy issues that affect physician receptivity to CQI can be discussed from a number of perspectives. One of the most useful is to examine these issues from the perspectives of physicians themselves. Properly interpreted, physicians' perceptions of the way the outside world affects their lives constitute concrete and immediate data on the forces that make it easier and harder for them to participate in efforts to improve quality of care. One source of such data with which we have particular familiarity is the attitudes and beliefs of the membership of the ACP, which represents the nation's practitioners of internal medicine.

The membership of the ACP seems most concerned with four general areas at the current time. First is the redistribution of power in the health care system, which is manifested most directly in the changing governance or ownership of health plans. Whether one is discussing health maintenance organizations, multispecialty clinics, single specialty groups, or other arrangements, the way an organization is controlled and the nature of its ownership are extremely important because governance and ownership are vital influences on the goals of a health care organization. ACP members want to know particularly whether the new organizational forms in health care—integrated health care delivery systems and other large arrangements controlled by insurance companies or other investors—will share the same goals physicians traditionally have pursued. To what extent will administrators of such organizations strive to maximize profit, and will conflict arise between profit maximization and the preservation of physician autonomy? Will physicians be micromanaged to reduce health care use? Will new financial incentives in such companies drive a wedge between doctors and their patients?

Obviously, physicians' level of trust in the goals and values of the organizations for which they increasingly work will play a critical role in determining their receptivity to the management priorities of those organizations. Management necessarily is involved in the adoption and implementation of TQM. Indeed, some of the work discussed elsewhere in this volume suggests that organizational leaders must be personally and heavily committed to TQM if it is to work. Unfortunately, when physicians mistrust the ownership of a health care institution, they may greet even the more positive initiatives of that organization with skepticism and suspicion.

A second area of major concern to ACP members is malpractice. One of the authors (JRB) has been involved in assessing malpractice and defensive medicine for almost twenty-five years. Policymakers have traditionally underestimated the psychological effect on physicians of the malpractice threat that hangs over them. For example, at a recent presentation on health reform Ball made to a group of physicians' spouses, the only spontaneous applause occurred in response to comments on the need to strengthen malpractice reform. That example emphasizes the powerful negative force the malpractice threat has on physicians. This threat, in turn, affects how physicians view quality improvement.

In general, physicians come from a culture that requires them to make life-and-death decisions for which they are solely responsible. The socialization of physicians emphasizes personal accountability in both large and small ways. A common refrain in residency training is "If you want to be sure it's done right, do it yourself!" This sense of personal responsibility and accountability is multiplied many times by the certain knowledge that if something goes wrong during the care of a patient and a suit results, the physician will be a target of that suit, regardless of the reason for the original problems.

The quality improvement movement, in contrast, emphasizes quite appropriately that modern health care organizations have become enormously complex webs of interconnecting processes that depend on teamwork and interpersonal communication to function effectively. Delegation and sharing of tasks and information are crucial to quality. Physicians are dependent on other workers whether they like it or not and are far better off when they recognize and take advantage of such dependencies. Thus, the reality of modern health care processes and the teaching of TQM run directly counter to the message conveyed not only by physicians' training but also by public policy acting through our tort system.

A third policy issue for ACP members is the volume and use of information. One concern that members have is how they can master the enormous amount of information that is relevant to their work. Each year, about four million articles are published in twenty-nine thousand journals in the medical literature alone. No one individual can stay abreast of this volume of material, much less adapt it intelligently to daily practice.

But a second and even more troubling information-related concern for physicians is the increasing use of data for what they perceive to be hostile purposes: to monitor and, perhaps, to discipline them. The initial release of Medicare hospital mortality data by the Health Care Financing Administration (HCFA) was strongly opposed by the American Medical Association, the American Hospital Association, and others. More recent examples of similar use of data have occurred in New York and Pennsylvania. Physicians worry that hospital and managed care administrators will either use such data on clinical performance incorrectly— drawing premature or insupportable conclusions—or use it for purposes that physicians oppose, such as economic credentialing.

A critical precondition for the effective implementation of the methods of TQM is that members of any organization must be willing to share data about performance with the organization's physicians. Without such willingness, quality problems cannot be accurately diagnosed or addressed. The current rush to collect and publicly release data about physician performance is making it increasingly difficult to enlist physicians in TQM activities.

The fourth policy issue of concern to ACP members is that changing financial incentives are creating new conflicts between physicians' financial interests and their patients' wishes. In the current fee-for-service system, physicians believe that their financial incentives usually are aligned fairly closely with their patients' preferences: when a patient needs or wants a procedure, the physician gets financially rewarded for doing it. This same physician may feel pressure from society to conserve resources, but at least the patient and the physician generally think and act along parallel paths. Under many managed care arrangements, however, physicians get paid for doing less. Although some experts may regard this arrangement as better for quality of care, it is not clear yet that patients have embraced the idea that less is better. As the realization spreads that physicians benefit financially by reducing services to patients, the possibility of resentment and conflict between patient and physician grows. This possibility is personally disturbing to those physicians who find gratification in a trusting patient-physician relationship. From the standpoint of quality management, such conflicts between the physician—the supplier—and the patient—the customer—are also destructive to the customer-supplier relationships that are essential to CQI. TQM emphasizes that long-term and trusting partnerships between customers and suppliers create conditions in which customers can communicate their needs effectively and suppliers can refine their processes of production to meet those needs as precisely as possible. A health care system in which patients and physicians eye each other with suspicion and mistrust would be anathema to TQM.

Each of these four policy issues needs attention if physicians are to be engaged more meaningfully in CQI: (1) the changing ownership and control of health care organizations and the resulting implications for alignment of goals between physicians and the institutions for which they increasingly work, (2) the threat of medical malpractice and its effect on physicians' willingness to share responsibility in ways that are required to make CQI effective, (3) the increasing perception among physicians that information can be harmful to their well-being as practitioners, a perception that is poisonous to data-based quality improvement, and (4) the consequences of changing financial incentives in the health care system for the patient-physician relationship.

Changing Physician Behavior

Even if all of the above-mentioned policy issues were addressed, the effort to engage physicians in CQI would have to tackle the age-old question of how one gets physicians to change their behavior. To find the answer to this conundrum, one needs to know more about how physicians currently make decisions and what factors are likely to affect such decisions.

Information is clearly one influence on physician behavior, but the manner and strength of its influence remain matters of some dispute. It is commonly reported that only about 10 percent of what clinicians do is supported by scientific evidence from randomized controlled clinical trials or other studies. As previously noted, the volume of information is such that, even where it exists, many physicians find it difficult to assimilate.

We believe that five factors are necessary to change physician behavior. The first factor is data, and they must be valid data. The second factor is a credible source of those data. If, for example, the Health Care Financing Administration (HCFA) published guidelines on the proper way to treat cholecystitis, nobody would believe them. If, however, the Agency for Health Care Policy and Research (AHCPR) published similar guidelines, the chance of acceptance by physicians would be better. Similarly, if the Centers for Disease Control and Prevention (CDCP) published a guideline for influenza immunization, everyone would use it because of the credibility of the source.

The third factor necessary to change physician behavior is appropriate incentives for physicians to use information. For many years, the ACP has produced clinical guidelines. By themselves, however, they are not followed, even if they are published in a credible journal. For years, the National Institutes of Health (NIH) has run consensus development conferences that pull together the best available information on controversial clinical topics. The results are published and publicized. Yet, studies have demonstrated that only 1 percent of physicians generally are aware of the existence of any particular consensus development conference, can identify any of its recommendations, and actually follow particular prescriptions. Making available valid information from a credible source does not make a difference without a corresponding incentive to use that information. And, although there are many other reasons why physicians do things, among the most powerful are financial incentives. Consequently, the ACP has been working with the Blue Cross and Blue Shield Associations during the last seventeen years to include clinical guidelines designed to change clinical behavior in Blue Cross/Blue Shield payment policies.

Until recently, these three factors seemed sufficient to potentiate change in physician behavior. However, two more factors now also appear to be important. The first of these is a safe environment. For reasons discussed above—physicians' suspicion of the motives of health plans, their fear of malpractice, and their worry that government and other forces are watching their every move with hostile intent—the current practice environment certainly does not feel safe for physicians trying to use information. Until that environment is made safe, it is unlikely that CQI will flourish. It is incumbent upon all who work in the health care arena to promote changes that will make the practice environment safe for doctors without sacrificing appropriate and necessary mechanisms to ensure the accountability of professionals.

The final factor necessary to promote modifications in physician behavior is a cultural change that necessarily will have to start in medical schools. In general, physicians are not team players, in part, because they are selected for their individual academic excellence much more than their ability to work with others and, in part, because of the way they are indoctrinated throughout the educational process. The concept of true teamwork needs to be fostered from the start of medical education. It needs to be emphasized in students' initial patient care experiences and communicated by residents to interns and faculty to residents. Teamwork needs to be integrated into the concept of professionalism. Without this cultural change, we cannot really have CQI.

Thus, five factors are necessary to promote change in physician behavior: (1) valid information from (2) a credible source, (3) incentives to use that information, (4) a safe practice environment, and ultimately, (5) a cultural change in the profession of medicine.

Some Personal Experiences with Quality Improvement

To some degree, these perceptions of the requirements for changing physician behavior reflect the authors' personal experiences and observations over the years with public and private initiatives to improve quality of care. We share these here with the hope of making some of these lessons more vivid. Another conclusion from this experience is that even under ideal circumstances, getting physicians to champion the cause of TQM will be a formidable task. And yet, such leadership will prove essential to the success of CQI over the long term.

1. Professional Standards Review Organizations. The Professional Standards Review Organizations (PSRO) program was created by Congress in the early 1970s for the purpose of containing the costs and improving the quality of care under the federal Medicare program. The PSRO program was the precursor to the existing Peer Review Organization (PRO) program that HCFA currently operates.

In the early years of the PSRO program, one of its objectives was to refine quality assurance techniques through so-called medical care evaluation studies. Medical care evaluation studies used a ten-step protocol that began by identifying a meaningful problem and then moved to develop criteria by which the problem would be measured, extract charts, find variations from the charts, explain the variation, put a treatment plan in place, and reevaluate what had been accomplished. At the time, it seemed a logical and scientific approach to quality improvement, and indeed it has many similarities to the PDCA (plan-do-check-act) cycle advocated under current theories of CQI. However, medical care evaluation studies did not catch on at all. Why? The simplest explanation is that the process was not well received because it was developed and demanded by parties external to the profession. Even though the authors of the legislation intended to give control *to* the profession of medicine, professionals never accepted the PSRO program, in part, probably because it was not *from* medicine. If history is any guide, for quality improvement efforts to work, they must involve physicians from the start.

2. Medicare Coverage Policy. Another early quality-related experiment was the process for setting health care coverage policy for Medicare. It is a little known fact that the Medicare legislation provides virtually no guidance to the HCFA concerning which technologies are legitimate services under Medicare and which tests and treatments are not legitimate and, therefore, not deserving of coverage. To understand the importance and difficulty of coverage policy questions, consider that Medicare historically has been required to make all of the decisions that private insurers have had to make about which technologies to pay for: heart, liver, and bone marrow transplantation; new cancer drugs and new AIDS treatments; and so on.

Given the complexity of such coverage determinations and the billions of dollars involved for the federal government, one might imagine that HCFA would have devoted considerable resources to the effort. Wrong. In the early 1970s, the entire staff for the task consisted of one secretary and one physician who were given no external medical supervision and no regulatory guidance to aid in decision making. The only directive came from the Medicare law itself: that Medicare should not pay for things that were not necessary for the care and treatment of disease.

The first issue the coverage policy project had to address was computed tomography of the body: CT scans. Without a defensible process by which to make a recommendation, and without anything like sufficient data on which to base a recommendation, the office was unable to give effective coverage advice to the Medicare program. Later, Congress legislated the creation of the National Center for Health Care Technology (NCHCT) in 1978, which inherited the responsibility for making coverage decisions. This new entity had a very modest appropriation and an advisory council: it wasn't perfect, but it was a big step forward from the ad hoc process that preceded it. However, the NCHCT ran into its own problems. One problem was the budget cutbacks of the early days of the Reagan administration. A second problem was the opposition of the medical profession as conveyed by the American Medical Association (AMA). Staff at the NCHCT, anticipating the current role of the AHCPR, sought to develop guidelines, standards, and norms on how technology should be approached. This development threatened the perceived autonomy of health professionals. Once again, the profession rallied to reject a quality improvement effort that came from outside its own ranks. The NCHCT lost its appropriation in 1981, three years after it was created, and only recently have its functions been revived in anything like the original form.

3. *Clinical Efficacy Assessment Project.* A third experience with early application of quality improvement technology in health care was with the Clinical Efficacy Assessment Project of the ACP, which was organized in the early 1980s. Through this project, the ACP assessed individual technologies and asked what the data revealed about their appropriate use. We attempted to enable physicians to base their practice behavior on data more than on habit or anecdote. The process the ACP developed was fairly advanced for the early 1980s, and as part of this process, we attempted to get other physician organizations involved. From 1981 to 1984, however, representatives of most other physician organizations in internal medicine refused to become involved, in part, because they were afraid of being sued and, in part, because they did not want to appear directive to their membership.

The ACP persisted, nonetheless, and this process has become a valuable endeavor. In fact, people now think that practice parameters and guidelines are worthwhile. The early opposition, though, provided yet another example of resistance to the threat of diminished professional autonomy.

4. Hospitals and Physicians. During the last several years, one of us (JRB) also has had the opportunity to look at what hospitals and physicians are doing in quality improvement from the perspective of a judge in the Health Care Forum/Witt Quality Award. To receive this award, hospital administrators nominated their organizations themselves. Strikingly, in nearly every hospital, the physician side of the quality improvement effort was always separate from the administrative side. The two almost never got together. In addition, the applicants for the award and the people pushing CQI within these hospitals uniformly came from the administrative side. An application was never generated by the physician professional community, although logically, physicians should have been at the forefront. This same finding has been manifest in another national program aimed at promoting quality of care in hospitals: the Robert Wood Johnson Foundation project on hospital quality improvement. Again, leadership in quality improvement comes from the hospital administrators, not physicians.

In all four of these examples, one might have thought and hoped that physicians would have had interest in quality improvement. As physicians, we should be in the business of continually improving our practice and our patient outcomes, but within the quality improvement movement, we typically have not assumed leadership.

What can be learned from such experiences? In general, they do not particularly cast physicians in the light of Jeffersonian creatures—hungry for information and prompt to respond and to do the right thing. The resistance of physicians to change is obviously deep-seated, and their suspicion of outside efforts to promote change is profound. Resolving the policy issues discussed above and lining up the necessary forces to promote change in physician behavior may or may not be sufficient to achieve the results that ultimately are needed: joyful leadership by physicians to promote quality improvement.

American College of Physicians

The experience of the ACP may be instructive on where CQI may head in the future. Although none of the college's membership or the board or any of the staff think of the ACP this way, it is really a small business. The college has 280 employees, an annual budget of $40 million, and four product lines: publications, a set of educational programs, health and public policy development, and a membership organization and benefits.

In its early days, people joined the college because it was prestigious. Members received the denotation "Fellow, American College of Physicians"; they shared membership with elite physicians; and not everybody was accepted. The college developed excellent products, some of which were unique, such as the *Annals of Internal Medicine* and the *Medical Knowledge Self-Assessment Program*, and customers bought these products because they were unique and of high quality.

Now, the college is in a new phase: competition. Not all of our products are unique anymore. To survive and prosper, the college must not only represent its membership but also serve them as well. This dichotomy is a familiar problem for health care organizations in our newly competitive health care system.

These changes have forced the college to change in two respects. First, instead of being merely an honorific society or the producer of educational products, the college must be a real membership association; this means we must listen to the customer, the member. This is a concept that the board of the organization has not yet fully understood and that the staff has not yet fully accepted.

Second, the college is forced to deal with the requirement to provide truly excellent service. With this goal in mind, it formed a customer service unit and started to collect data. The ACP received 20,000 phone calls a month, and in one year had 229,000 individual transactions with its members. It was able to divide these transactions into sixteen categories to get some normative data on how long certain transactions were taking, to set some standards on how long they ought to take and on how many people could be expected to be dropped from telephone calls, and how long different phone calls should require. As a result, the ACP brought about a one-stop shopping service that made sense as a business strategy. Some staff, however, had not fully bought into the new approach. Those most against it were the program people, who questioned the allocation of resources to customer service.

The college exists because of its members, its customers. Reorienting the college's culture to be sensitive to needs of those customers has been painful and slow, but by applying different measurement techniques and demonstrating value, both internal and external, this reorientation process has begun to work.

Another way to help change the organization's culture is to use staff evaluation methods with creativity. For most staff, evaluation is made on the basis of individual performance, but the college has begun to add performance evaluations of team participation: did the individual participate in team activities? Did the team do well? Not surprisingly, individuals are initially somewhat leery about being evaluated, in part, by what somebody else does (the team), and they are especially sensitive to the issue of whether a raise will depend—even in part—on that team performance evaluation.

At the college are five very senior physician managers. For these managers, evaluation has consisted of three facets: (1) how did the college do, (2) how did the division do, and (3) how did the individual do? The evaluation rating is in that order with descending value. Notably, the new CEO of IBM recently stated a similar focus for IBM's senior management: your bonuses will be determined, not by how your division does, but by how all of IBM does. The ethic is: "We are all in this together." Thus, we need to change the organization's culture to demonstrate the importance of the whole.

Physicians at this point, having been trained to be individually responsible for life-and-death decisions and knowing that the threat of malpractice hangs over their heads, will find it very difficult to change their approaches to share responsibilities: "you mean I'm going to be responsible for what somebody else does that I can't control?" Predictably, resistance to change will be tremendous.

Discussion

To return to the policy issues that began this discussion, the first issue addressed was that of ownership in health systems. Physicians all have a responsibility to ensure that system ownership strives to serve the needs of human health first, rather than profits. Insurance companies and other investor-owned entities have a great advantage because they have capital, logical structures, and presumably, a spirit of entrepreneurship among managers.

The goal of a health system, however, must be to improve the health outcomes of people over time. Although physicians, for the most part, still have that as the principal goal, it remains to be seen whether the new economic entities that are increasingly dominating the health care landscape will share these values. There are clear cases in which profit making may run counter to good practice. Administrators of a prepaid health plan who are more interested in serving their investors than their patients would logically not be too interested in expensive population-based disease prevention exercises, such as hypertension education. The odds are that the benefits of such programs would not be realized for many years, and members may very well have moved on by then to other health care plans and will then be the beneficiaries of other plans' investments. It is uncertain whether administrators of insurance companies or existing HMOs will really promote this as their goal. We have a real responsibility to demand that—regardless of their ownership—the goal of whatever networks we construct is to improve the health outcomes of patients over time.

The second policy issue raised was malpractice. A major problem with the way the medical profession approaches the malpractice issue is that the forest is lost for the trees. Physicians still believe that simple tort reform and attacking lawyers' profits are sufficient. Instead, they should be supporting a no-fault approach. The work of the Harvard School of Public Health in Massachusetts has shown that if we had universal health coverage, we could cover health care misadventures through a no-fault malpractice system. Rather than use the blunt, ineffective tool of malpractice suits to batter physicians into line, other forms of quality interventions could be used to improve physician performance. The current system only serves to prevent physicians from making good clinical decisions almost every day while it creates a barrier to physician involvement in CQI. If our society could forget all the nonsense on malpractice and move to a no-fault system that really compensates people who are injured, we will have removed a major obstacle to securing cooperation of physicians in furthering the best interests of patients and the health care system overall.

Concerning the availability and use of information, it is encouraging that physicians and institutional leaders seem to be recognizing that it is to their benefit to produce data demonstrating the value of what they do. As an example, the managers of U.S. Health Care, a large HMO, recently threatened not to contract with Pennsylvania Hospital in Philadelphia for hip surgery even though Pennsylvania Hospital had one of the highest volumes of hip surgery in the nation. This threat to withdraw was prompted by the fact that charges and length of stays at Pennsylvania Hospital were more than 50 percent above the regional average. Hospital staff had a real incentive to change, and in three months, length of stay was decreased by 30 percent and charges by 50 percent.

As the health care system changes under health reform initiatives, physicians will face increased pressure to demonstrate the value of what they do. In fact, leaders at many organizations already show a real sense of pride in measuring and proving how well their enterprises are doing. Good physicians and good hospital executives will want to provide valid and clear information not only because it will enable them to compete more effectively but also because of this pride in excellence. Researchers and practitioners need to develop and disseminate the necessary tools to collect, interpret, and use such information.

Finally, returning to the fourth policy problem of misalignment of financial incentives facing physicians, here physicians face a real problem. This problem stems from the combined influence of physicians' habits and patients' expectations that are fueled by contact with a technologically fascinated society. How can physicians educate patients enough so that they understand that more is not always better? This will require a major societal change.

As physicians, we have a huge educational change to encourage among our patients. However, how can such a change occur when, with realigned financing, physicians will be paid more for doing less patient care while patients still believe that more is better? Outcomes research may help, but major educational programs are necessary to promote new alliances between patients and doctors.

Although the culture of physicians does not guarantee that physicians as a group are willing to change, the prospects for change are bright. Focusing on real problems and solutions encourages change in even the most resistant people, especially when, at heart, almost every physician means to do well. By providing physicians with information, the tools to change, and a just and safe environment within which to practice, the achievable results will most certainly include demonstrably effective—yes, cost-effective—and caring medicine.

11

Perspectives and Possibilities

David Blumenthal, M.D., M.P.P.

One purpose of this book has been to begin a process of building conceptual and verbal bridges between communities that share deeply felt, common goals—the improvement of human health and our health care system—and yet seem to have found communication difficult. On the one side are practicing physicians and the health services researchers who are, respectively, serving patients and working to improve the decision-making capability of physicians. On the other side are health care administrators and a devoted band of thinkers and quality practitioners who see total quality management (TQM) as important to improving the functioning of our health care system. These disparate groups work in and around the same institutions and customers and often participate in the same processes or struggle from the outside to improve them. The underlying assumptions and methods they use in their work are overlapping and synergistic. Yet, they often eye each other with skepticism.

These attitudes may be a passing anomaly of the early years of a profound revolution in quality management within our health care system. If so, the premise that motivated this volume may have been faulty. However, that is not important. The important thing is that the relevant communities fully explore the possibilities for quality improvement that may be realized if and when physicians and health services researchers, on the one hand, and advocates of continuous quality improvement (CQI), on the other, work together.

From the standpoint of the physician, the most important such opportunities lie in at least two general areas: (1) the potential to enhance the scientific basis of daily medical practice and, relatedly, (2) the potential to enhance the professionalism of medicine and consumer faith in physicians at a time when both professionalism and the physician-patient relationship are under extraordinary stress. The purpose of this chapter is to explore further both the potential value of applying the tools of modern quality management to patient management and the nature of the obstacles confronting this effort.

Enhancing the Scientific Basis of Practice

Since the release of the Flexner Report in 1911[1], those in the profession of medicine have striven to ground their practice in the scientific method. Physicians' faith in their own craft rests to a substantial degree on what they see as the scientific underpinnings of their work. And as Starr[2] indicated, the public's faith in physicians also depends on the perception that physicians have access to and strive to apply a body of scientifically valid information about health and disease. Recognizing the importance of science to medical practice, instructors at medical schools provide students with a healthy dose of basic biological science—biochemistry, physiology, genetics, pathophysiology, molecular biology, microbiology—and with at least some exposure to analytical methods (experimental design and statistical analysis) so that they can continue to appreciate the medical literature after they leave medical school. Curricula of most residency programs support this orientation by requiring that residents and interns learn to use the medical literature and to appraise it critically.

The public, too, has played an underappreciated but essential role in maintaining the scientific basis of medical practice. This role has consisted chiefly of unwavering support during the last fifty years for the funding of biomedical research with taxpayers' money at the federal and state level. The public, through its elected representatives, also has insisted in recent years that the new knowledge generated by this research be translated promptly into practice[3] so that the practicing physician and their patients can have access to it as rapidly as possible.

The shared commitment of physicians and the public to promoting the scientific basis of medical practice has served them both well over time. Although some experts legitimately criticize what they perceive as excessive reliance on new technologies generated by the research establishment, there is little doubt that the rigor of medical training and standards of practice in the United States are unexcelled anywhere in the world.

And yet, the scientific legitimacy of American medicine is far from secure at the current time. As Blendon[4] and Donelan[5] noted, the public's faith in the profession has plummeted during the last thirty years. In 1966, fully 73 percent of Americans had a great deal of confidence in the leaders of American medicine, compared with 20 percent in 1994. The reasons for this decline in confidence are multiple, but one factor seems to be the growing evidence, highlighted by Mulley in this volume (see Chapter Four), of unexplained variations in medical practice and outcomes of care in the United States. Such variations graphically expose what many physicians must reluctantly admit: despite the accomplishments of medical science, only a small proportion of the interventions they undertake in daily practice actually are supported by valid scientific data. Even more troubling is the evidence cited by Ball (see Chapter Ten) that when such information exists, the practicing American physician is frequently unaware of it. This lack of awareness creates great uncertainty among physicians about what to do when presented with common and uncommon medical problems.

Inconsistency, variation in practice, and variation in outcome thrive in the presence of such uncertainty. The variation phenomenon is not about the evil or incompetence of doctors; it is about the persistent inadequacy of the science base informing medical practice—an inadequacy resulting from gaps in knowledge and failures in systems for disseminating existing knowledge.

One very revealing phenomenon highlights the disconnection between practicing physicians and the scientific process that has contributed to their legitimacy with the public. This phenomenon is the fact that so few physicians participate in systematic experimentation to learn from their daily patient experience. One important reason for this lack is that research techniques have become so sophisticated in the modern era that advanced training and expensive logistical support are required to conduct clinical investigation that is considered valid by the experts who review results for funding and publication. The very elementary exposure to experimental and analytical methods that most physicians receive in medical school is no longer adequate. The process of learning from clinical practice, therefore, now occurs almost exclusively in academic medical centers. The average physician's only contact with the process of discovery occurs when he or she reads journals or attends continuing education courses. Even those who might be interested in applying scientific principles to learning from their personal experience are led to understand that such experimentation is infeasible.

At least two consequences flow from physicians' lack of involvement in clinical experimentation. First, their ability to interpret scientific information conveyed from other sources erodes over time. Second, the information generated from their practices is never captured by the profession. After all, every time a physician diagnoses or treats a patient, a kind of experiment takes place that sheds light on the capability of the diagnostic or therapeutic method chosen. As Mulley noted, such information, were it captured, would provide an invaluable complement to clinical trials. Because they strive for scientific rigor, researchers in clinical trials often sacrifice relevance. Their findings apply directly only to the tiny percentage of patients who share the characteristics of subjects included in the trials.

Why is this review of the role of science in the daily practice of medicine helpful to the current discussion? To answer this question, it is useful to recall very briefly a point made earlier in this volume about the origins and purposes of TQM.

The body of knowledge now associated with TQM has evolved during eighty years of application in a variety of large settings, mostly large organizations. The original founders of the field of modern quality management were statisticians and engineers who had very practical goals. They wanted to reduce the number of defective telephones coming off the production lines of a manufacturing plant. Their work proceeded along two paths. Some of them worked on developing statistical methods for increasing the efficiency of quality monitoring. These new methods gave rise to what is now known as sampling theory. Another group of quality innovators took an even more practical tack. They set to work trying to make the statistical methods developed by their colleagues into a tool kit that could be used by the types of people employed in industrial plants. After all, the point of the entire exercise was not to make conceptual breakthroughs, but to reduce the number of defective telephones sent to customers.

From the very beginning, therefore, TQM has had both a scientific and a very practical orientation. The scientific orientation has its foundation in statistical methods, engineering, and operations research. The practical orientation has been forced on the field by the customers whom it has tried to serve. These customers included, over time, not only industrial concerns but also the U.S. armed forces. During World War II, a number of the founders of TQM went to work in the proving grounds of the U.S. military with the job of improving the quality of U.S. armaments, which were often unreliable during the early years of the war.

Interestingly, the requirement to produce results and the commitment to scientific methods have been mutually reinforcing and have honed the tools of modern quality management over time. Methods of analysis that lack validity are unlikely to be useful over the long term. The practical orientation of TQM pushed its proponents to search broadly for techniques of quality improvement, and in the process, they uncovered methods and approaches that anticipated many of those applied by modern health services researchers to quality assurance in health care.

Outcome Measurement

Proponents of TQM have a fanatical commitment to measuring quality. They believe it is difficult or impossible to improve quality unless its critical attributes can be quantified. Definitions of quality vary in the TQM literature, but in all cases, the consumer is viewed as the ultimate arbiter. To measure quality without taking the customer's views into account in deciding what to measure is viewed as self-defeating because it is the customer's reaction that will determine the marketability of the product. Outcome measurement in health services research can be seen in many ways as consistent with the application of principles pioneered in industrial quality management to the sphere of health services. The effects of health care on health status (outcomes of care) are one dimension of quality. A major thrust of outcomes research—to identify and measure outcomes that are valued by patients—is perfectly consistent with TQM as it has been practiced by industrial organizations during the last eighty years.

Learning from Variation

Statisticians love variation for what it has to teach about the behavior of the world around them. It was only natural, therefore, that the statisticians who pioneered industrial quality methods should focus on variation in outcomes and processes of production as a window on how those processes functioned and how outcomes could be improved. The statistical founders of TQM came eventually to view variation in some instances as dangerous to quality but also taught that variation was inevitable in both process and out-come and should not be misinterpreted. In particular, they pointed out the potential damage to quality that could be done by "tam-pering"—reacting to normal variation in a stable process as though it were abnormal and needed fixing. The result would be a deteri-oration in quality. The current interest in variation in health care processes and outcomes can be seen as the recognition among health services researchers that variation is important to quality in health care processes and outcomes, just as it is in industrial con-cerns. Many of the tools for studying variation and controlling it that have been introduced in industrial quality management are likely to prove useful in health care settings as well. Of particular note in this regard is Shewhart's control chart, discussed by Blu-menthal (see Chapter Two).

Exploratory Data Analysis (EDA)

Some of the tools introduced by industrial quality management for studying variation in processes and outcomes can be viewed as applications of what statisticians have called "exploratory data analysis" (EDA). Such techniques constitute the front line or trip wire of the quality monitoring process in industry. They are sim-ple methods for displaying and interpreting data so that patterns of interest can be discerned. Among the techniques of EDA used by TQM are stem and leaf plots, box plots, scatter diagrams, his-tograms and Pareto diagrams, and control charts. EDA is a rapid approach for turning data into information. Like a screening test in medicine, its techniques are sensitive and suggestive but not spe-cific or definitive.

The use of EDA by industrial quality managers has been the source of some misunderstanding. As Greenfield suggests (see Chap-ter Three), the screening tests applied to understand variation in industrial processes sometimes are interpreted by health services researchers as a sign of the statistical naivete of practitioners of TQM. Rather, properly used, EDA serves to inform the development of hypotheses that can be tested with more rigorous statistical analysis of existing data or through formal experimentation. EDA is a way to screen hypotheses for testing, an essential step in the real world because the number of possible causes of any particular quality problem is often so large as to make assessing them all impractical.

Guideline Development

Among the tools used for quality improvement is a technique called the flowchart. A *flowchart* consists of boxes and arrows that describe explicitly the steps in industrial processes that result in the transformation of inputs to outputs. Such flowcharts are used in several ways: as diagnostic tools to reveal unnecessary repetition that causes waste, inefficiency, and poor quality; as analytical devices to assist in the redesign of processes; as tools for teaching revised processes to workers; and as monitoring devices for making certain that improved processes continue to be followed. Flowcharts thus serve both analytical and prescriptive purposes. The guidelines, algorithms, and critical paths now advocated in health care settings are virtually identical in appearance to industrial flowcharts. Change the medical terminology to manufacturing jargon, and the identity becomes perfect. Furthermore, guidelines/flowcharts are coming to serve almost identical functions in health care as they have served in industrial quality management. A good example is the use of guidelines by Park Nicollet Clinic in Minneapolis (see Chapter Nine). Physicians and administrators at Park Nicollet used flowcharts of the original process for diagnosing breast masses to identify problems in that process. They then revised the protocol, formulated a new flowchart (guideline), and disseminated it in a newsletter in order to educate other physicians.

Survey Research to Improve Quality Management

Although it is not widely discussed, W. Edwards Deming, one of the founders of modern industrial quality management, spent most of the 1940s perfecting techniques of survey research.[6] During the early part of that decade, he worked for the U.S. Bureau of the Census, helping its surveyors improve their sampling methods. When he traveled to Japan in the early 1950s—to help initiate Japan's quality revolution—his nominal mission was to assist American occupation administrators with the development and implementation of the first postwar census of the Japanese population. Perhaps Deming's personal experience had something to do with an enduring characteristic of modern industrial quality management: a strong commitment to the use of survey techniques to ascertain the views of consumers and to apply those views to perfecting products and processes for producing those products. In recent years, the world of health care quality has placed increasing emphasis on the use of surveys of patients to provide information on the quality of care and service and to guide efforts to improve processes of care.[7,8] This emphasis has given rise to the concept of "patient-centered care." Here again, the potential utility of valid, reliable data on patient's views of quality was anticipated by developments in industrial quality management.

The reason for drawing out the multiple ways in which TQM's methods foreshadowed those of modern health services research is not to glorify the former or to underestimate the contributions of the latter. Rather, the point is this: practitioners of industrial quality management developed and used these technologies for quality improvement because they understood the scientific method, were devoted to its use, and spent eighty years trying to apply it in daily work. Outcomes measurement, the study of variation, EDA, guidelines, survey research, and other techniques of TQM are simply the logical and inevitable outgrowth of such science-based efforts to improve the capabilities of workers and organizations endeavoring to serve the needs of large groups of customers in a complicated, changing world. The founders of industrial quality management and TQM got to these techniques earlier than health services research because they shared a similar worldview, similar aims, and started half a century sooner.

A number of conclusions would seem to flow naturally from this understanding of the history and development of industrial quality management science. Given TQM's long effort to bring scientific methods to bear on processes of service and production, and given the similarities of its technologies to those now under development in health care quality management, the possibility exists that TQM may provide a prepackaged, tried and tested bag of tools and tricks for improving quality of clinical care by bringing scientific methods to bear on daily practice. If that is the case—even if the possibility that it could prove true is remote—then it would make sense for physicians and health services researchers interested in improving health care quality to pore over every text and treatise on industrial quality management in the hope that a few useful nuggets would be discovered. It also would make sense for those techniques, once uncovered, to be taught to medical students and physicians in training so that they could use them to improve continuously the quality of care they provide. In the process, it may turn out that the field of industrial quality management also has much to learn from the tools and approaches currently under development by health services researchers.

Were the techniques of TQM to prove useful in augmenting science-based decision making in clinical practice, a number of benefits might flow from this development. First and foremost, the quality of care provided to the average patient might improve. Second, physicians might be empowered to derive useful information from their daily practice, just as TQM empowers industrial workers to learn from their daily work. As noted in Chapter Two, TQM provides tools for conducting valid experiments on processes without interrupting or disrupting them. Physicians currently conduct such experiments all the time. They think of it as "trial and error" and use their experience of patients' reactions to drugs and treatments to titrate those interventions. Rarely, however, do they apply statistically sound analytical methods to the appreciation of the experimental data derived from individual patient care. Neuhauser and his colleagues (see Chapter Five) show how simple tools taught by

TQM may allow physicians to derive more valid and reliable conclusions from the data generated by the response of individual patients to their medical regimens. The cumulative experience of physicians using such analytical techniques could provide insights into the process of care that would not otherwise have become available. This information would contribute to the goal, described by Mulley (see Chapter Four), of finding ways to learn constantly from the outcomes of clinical experience for the purpose of improving it.

Third, augmenting science-based decision making in modern medicine might assist in reviving public faith in the profession of medicine by helping medical professionals meet the public's expectations of medical professionals. Among those expectations are that physicians have access to scientifically sound information about health and disease and *apply that information correctly to the particular cases of individual patients*. It is necessary but not sufficient for physicians to understand the latest information flowing from our nation's biomedical research. Physicians must be able to take that information and apply it logically, rationally, and appropriately to the treatment regimens they design for each of their patients. To accomplish this requires valid methods for learning from daily experience, for turning the data of patient care into information for decision making. TQM may be uniquely suited to meeting this challenge and, thereby, to enhancing public faith in the capabilities of medical professionals and the profession's faith in itself.

Barriers to Introducing TQM into Clinical Practice

To realize the full potential of this interaction between TQM and the work of clinical care and health services research, several barriers must be overcome. Perhaps the most formidable is a cultural gap between "TQMers" and physicians. To make the scientific method appealing to workers and managers with little experience or understanding of it, the practitioners of industrial quality management techniques have modified their message over time. This modification reflects very directly the experience of founders of TQM who discovered that more direct attempts to interest managers and workers in statistical and experimental methods as approaches to quality improvement were unsuccessful. For years, Deming tried to spread modern quality methods by teaching courses on statistics. He got nowhere.[6] So, he substituted an inspirational and motivational message to try to engage the imagination and commitment of managers and workers and boiled down the complex teachings of TQM to his "fourteen points," which could be listed on one side of a page. The exhortatory tone of TQM has infected the rhetoric of later generations of quality consultants, who, not surprisingly, have come to be viewed as "disciples" of the founding fathers of the quality movement.

Judging by the considerable success of the modern quality movement in Japan and now in U.S. industry, the inspirational, quasi-religious tone of TQM has proven successful in breaking down resistance by many laypersons in large companies. At a minimum, the approach taken by TQMers has not created insuperable obstacles to the adoption of modern quality management techniques by many industrial organizations. The same may not prove true in health care, however, at least where physicians and health services researchers are concerned. Physicians and researchers tend to be skeptical of the value of cultural and psychological interventions as methods for changing organizations. Yet, TQM often presents itself at first blush as a kind of management cult that emphasizes first and foremost a transformation of norms and values as the key to improving quality. Teachers and writers in the TQM movement often talk of the importance of changing the culture of organizations, of putting quality first, of paradigm shifts, of accomplishing "the transformation," of finding "joy in work," and of the importance of leadership. Their message often is conveyed in anecdotes that sound like parables that might be used by proponents of Eastern religions.

It would be incorrect to see the inspirational message of TQM as purely cosmetic. Anyone who has tried, as a manager or leader, to motivate large numbers of individuals to work together for organizational or civic purposes will understand the critical importance of a guiding idea or vision and of the value system, mission, and culture of an organization or a citizenry in achieving common purposes, including quality improvement.

However, few physicians and researchers have had the experience of trying to manage or lead other men and women or even of working in large groups or institutions. Physicians' scientific training, together with their individualism and lack of organizational exposure, makes them unreceptive and even hostile to the transformational vision of TQM. New approaches will have to be developed for enlisting the energetic cooperation of physicians and researchers in efforts to introduce CQI into health care organizations.

Those methods are now under development in leading health care institutions. Some promising approaches and associated problems are discussed by Shortell and his colleagues (Chapter Eight) and by Blumenthal and Edwards (Chapter Nine). Physicians are more likely to understand and support CQI efforts when they are motivated by valid and reliable data documenting problems with current performance, when they address clinical problems that physicians regard as important to patients, when they produce clinically meaningful changes in the process and outcomes of care, when they do not require physicians to sacrifice income or impose undue burdens on their colleagues, and when the improvement efforts are led by physician opinion leaders within their organizations or groups. As more physicians come to work in organizations, their general receptivity to modern quality management methods also may increase.

As Shortell and his colleagues point out, however, these approaches to introducing quality improvement methods do not resolve an important dilemma for health care organizations. To the extent that strategy and vision are important to the success of TQM (and they almost certainly are), the aforementioned approaches to gaining physician cooperation may not be sufficient. Here, Ball's assertion (see Chapter Ten) that the socialization of physicians must involve greater attention to their role as members of a health care team rings especially true. It may be that the foundation for successful quality improvement in health care—at least so far as the physician is concerned—must be laid in the earliest days of medical schools and must be reinforced continuously throughout medical training.

A second important barrier to promoting cooperation and synergy between modern industrial quality methods and the work of physicians and health services researchers consists of the real differences between the process of delivering clinical care and the process of industrial production. Although these differences sometimes are overstated by skeptics of TQM, they are real and important and must be acknowledged if industrial quality methods are to be adapted successfully to clinical settings.

One basic difference between the clinical medicine and some industrial settings concerns the nature of the inputs to clinical and industrial processes. At least in manufacturing organizations, it is often possible, through diligent effort, to improve quality by reducing variability in, and by improving the quality of, the raw materials used in the production process. The better and less variable the silicon chips used in computers, the better the quality of the machine is likely to be. In contrast, the critical "input" to the clinical process—the patient—is highly and inevitably variable. Indeed, at least in the United States, that variability is prized and celebrated, and adapting to it is considered essential to quality of care.

Another fundamental difference between the clinical and industrial settings concerns the complexity of the biological processes with which clinicians must deal, compared with the industrial processes with which TQM has concerned itself heretofore. As every high school student learns in basic biology, many fundamental aspects of human biology remain mysterious. Human life is the culmination of billions of years of evolution. The most elementary processes by which humans nourish themselves, maintain vital functions, reproduce, experience pain and pleasure, and learn are exquisitely complex and are yielding only grudgingly to massive efforts to unravel them. Industrial processes, in contrast, are human creations that have achieved their current level of complexity only in the last few decades of human evolution. As human creations, they often have blueprints to explain them. When they do not, they can be observed from the outside and analyzed. At least in theory, industrial processes can be stopped, disassembled, and reassembled in order to understand them better and to iron out problems that affect quality. Auto plants can be closed for "retooling." The medical profession cannot close its doors to reconfigure the biological processes of health and disease.

Physicians are correct, therefore, in arguing that clinical care is fraught with uncertainties that may not face managers of industrial quality. However, just because differences exist in the underlying processes of clinical medicine and manufacturing, it does not follow logically that the tools used to improve quality in one setting are completely inapplicable to the other. In fact, a close examination of the industrial and clinical settings will reveal important similarities, as well as differences; and even where differences exist, the analytical methods used for industrial quality management still may provide valuable insight into how to improve clinical quality.

The analogies between the problems facing clinicians and industrial managers occur at many levels, and a number were explored earlier in this volume. At the most basic level are the similarities between how clinicians are taught to think about their patients' biological processes and how industrial managers think about industrial processes. In daily work, both clinicians and managers conceptualize the processes with which they are concerned (to the extent that they formally model them at all) as linear flows subject to internal and external controls. These models often may be simplistic, but they guide decision making in daily work and can be extremely useful in both clinical and industrial settings. The similarity in underlying models of key processes creates opportunities to explore the application of industrial quality control technologies to the management of individual patients.

Similarly, important analogies exist between what physicians actually do to and with patients and the way industrial processes work. This is most clearly the case for elective surgical interventions or elective diagnostic or therapeutic procedures. Much of medicine starts with patients who are basically healthy but have an isolated problem or potential problem (for example, an inflamed appendix, a broken leg, gallbladder stones, a blocked artery in the heart, a headache, a sore back). These patients then are subjected to highly routinized, predictable, and focused interventions to investigate, ameliorate, or cure the problem. Such clinical interventions proceed, like basic industrial processes, according to well-defined blueprints. The processes are observable and analyzable and, therefore, potentially subject to the techniques used to improve industrial processes. James's application of TQM techniques to understanding the care of patients undergoing transurethral prostatectomy (see Chapter Seven) illustrates the application of TQM to such routinized interventions. Of course, there are always exceptions. Patients with coexisting illnesses or special anatomical problems require that processes be varied somewhat to meet their needs. Each physician may do things slightly differently from his or her colleagues. But the great majority of cases—particularly for a particular physician in a particular institution—proceed with remarkable predictability.

At still another level, physicians may find value in identifying opportunities to apply industrial quality methods to clinical problems that would seem, on first examination, to be fundamentally different from those encountered in industry. Mulley (Chapter Four) notes that clinical care can be seen as consisting of two distinct activities: (1) choosing a course of diagnosis or therapy and (2) executing the chosen intervention. Quality requires both choosing the right thing to do and doing the right thing right: decision quality and performance quality. A superficial review of TQM's applicability to clinical care might prompt the conclusion that techniques derived from industry would be relevant primarily to improving performance quality because diagnostic or treatment regimens have the most obvious similarities to industrial processes. Particularly in elective situations with stable, uncomplicated patients, the execution of such regimens has a mechanical and repetitive quality that resembles a manufacturing process.

In contrast, quality management methods used in industry would seem much less relevant to the activity of deciding what to do for a patient. Decision making is an intellectual, not a mechanical, activity. It is not observable or as easily analyzable as a treatment regimen. Furthermore, the decision-making process is variable, and appropriately so. Choosing the correct course of diagnosis or therapy involves a complicated interaction between patient and physician. The physician must ascertain the patient's preferences and tailor treatment to the unique needs and wishes of that individual. This procedure requires exchange of information in both directions. The decision-making process is the point at which treatment is customized and the individuality of the patient is made part of the treatment plan.

Nevertheless, the fact that physicians think of medical decision making as a process hints at possible opportunities to understand it better and even to improve it by using methods designed to improve industrial processes. This is the point at which most physicians begin to see TQM as threatening—anticipating that TQM will try to stamp out variability in decision making, just as it tries to stamp out variability in the execution of well-defined processes of production. However, a correct application of the principles of TQM might have just the opposite effect; it might enhance wanted variability while suppressing variability that is undesirable.

The key lies in TQM's dual concerns with meeting the needs and expectations of consumers (patients) and reducing variability in vital processes. If patients' needs and expectations differ, TQM would argue, then the process of care must vary as required to meet those needs and expectations. Otherwise, quality of care will be undermined. However, this does not mean the decision-making process itself should vary. Indeed, the outcome of that process is more likely to reflect the unique needs and expectations of patients if it is structured in a careful, methodical, and scientific way to elicit those expectations and to adapt the existing body of medical knowledge to them.

What does this mean in concrete terms? It means that as part of the process of diagnosing and treating illness, certain critical functions must be performed with a high degree of precision and regularity—that is, with a high level of quality. The patient must be given the information necessary to participate effectively in deciding what diagnostic or treatment option to pursue. The patient's expectations, needs, and values must be carefully and systematically elicited. The physician must be certain that he or she has access to all of the information relevant to this patient's problems: the patient's previous medical history, reactions to previous diagnostic and therapeutic interventions, the physician's personal experience with other similar patients, and the most recent medical literature on the patient's problems. The higher the quality with which these functions are performed, the more likely it is that the course of care will reflect the individuality of the patient—that desired variability will be preserved.

One way to achieve truly customized care is to reduce variability in the process of collecting and sharing the information required of appropriate decision making. This is, in essence, the purpose of the model of informed medical decision making envisioned by Mulley. Mulley envisions reducing variability in the processes that support decision making by using an interactive videodisc that provides the patient with impartial, understandable information and that elicits his or her preferences for alternative outcomes of care. In this way, variability attributable to the physician's personality, training, knowledge, style, and practice setting is reduced, and the patient is given an opportunity to receive and provide information that is valid, reliable, and appropriately tailored to the learning style and needs of that patient. Desired variability is preserved, while unwanted variability is reduced. The current effort to develop physician workstations (see Chapter Nine) that will give physicians access to the latest medical knowledge, including current guidelines for the use of diagnostic and therapeutic modalities, represents a similar attempt to reduce variability in processes by which physicians gather scientific information important to decision making.

By seeking ways to apply the lessons of TQM to clinical processes, other similar and potentially useful insights may emerge. Whether the application of TQM to the work of individual physicians and the process of clinical care will prove valuable will depend ultimately on empirical evidence concerning its utility. It is critical, however, that physicians and health services researchers approach this new body of knowledge with an open mind. It is also critical that proponents of TQM understand the culture of medicine and the special pressures and problems that confront the average medical practitioner, who constitutes, after all, an important customer of the quality improvement process. Only through diligent and unbiased effort will the quality of medical care be optimized in our health care system. Neither physicians nor health care managers can afford to leave any stone unturned in attempting to protect their craft, their patients, and their institutions as our health care system is radically transformed.

Notes

1. Flexner, A. (1910). *Medical Education in the U.S. and Canada* (Bulletin No. 4). New York: Carnegie Foundation for the Advancement of Teaching.

2. Starr, P. (1982). *The social transformation of American medicine*. New York: Basic Books.

3. Blumenthal, D. (1994). The vital role of professionalism in health care reform. *Health Affairs, 12*(1), 252–256.

4. Blendon, R. J. (1988). The public's view and the future of health care. *Journal of the American Medical Association, 259*, 3587–3593.

5. Donelan, K. (1994). *How do the needs of consumers play with managed care?* Paper presented at the Montgomery Dorsey Symposium. Beaver Creek, CO.

6. Walton, M. (1986). *The Deming management method.* New York: Putnam.

7. Cleary, P. D., Edgman-Leitan, S., Walker, J. D., Gerteis, M., Delbanco, T. I. (1993). Using patient reports to improve medical care: A preliminary report from 10 hospitals. *Quality Management in Health Care, 2*(91), 31–38.

8. Greenfield, S., Nelson, E. C. (1992). Recent developments and future issues in the use of health status assessment measures in clinical settings. *Medical Care, 30*(5 Suppl.), MS23–MS41.

Index

A

Ackoff, R., 11, 13
Acute care: blood pressure variability in, 152–159; statistical quality control (SQC) and, 40
Acute myocardial infarction (AMI) outcomes research case study, 60–64
Ambulatory blood pressure monitors, 144–146, 149–151
American College of Physicians (ACP), 276–277, 278–280
Angell, M., 182
Antihypertensive drugs, 149–151
Assignable variation, 189

B

Ball, J. R., 269, 277, 296
BCS (breast-conserving surgery), 85–86, 90, 93, 95–96
Benign prostatic hypertrophy (BPH). See Transurethral prostatectomy (TURP)
Berwick, D. M., 186, 234–235, 237
Blendon, R. J., 285
Blood pressure variability, 137–165; in acute care settings, 152–159; in ambulatory, clinically stable patients, 137–139, 151; ambulatory blood pressure monitors and, 144–146, 149–151; and assessing prognosis of hypertension, 147–149; control charts and, 156–157; defining, 139–141; and diagnosing hypertension, 146–147; diurnal blood pressure variations, 140–141; and measuring effects of antihypertensive drugs, 149–151; noninvasive measurement of, 143–146, 156; physiological control of blood pressure, 141–143; run charts and, 157–158; software for monitoring, 157–158; sphygmomanometers and, 143–144; total quality management (TQM) and, 138–139. See also Hypertension
Blumenthal, D., 238, 295

Box, G. E. P.: on control charts, 21; and evolutionary operations (EVOP), 43–44; on learning theory, 19
BPH (benign prostatic hypertrophy). See Transurethral prostatectomy (TURP)
Breast cancer outcomes research example, 81–96; breast-conserving surgery (BCS), 85–86, 90, 93, 95–96; estimating outcomes probabilities, 89–94; information needs and variation in decision making, 88–89, 97–101; mastectomies, 86, 90, 93, 95–96; outcome and practice variation and quality of care, 85–86; patient's decision-making role, 87–88; patient's perspective, 82–83; values, preferences, and controlling variation, 94–96. See also Outcomes research
Breast mass evaluation teams, 245–246

C

CABG (coronary artery bypass graft surgery), 83–85, 89–90, 91–92, 93–94, 95, 99
Case studies: acute myocardial infarction (AMI) outcomes research, 60–64; diabetes outcomes research, 65–67; Harvard Community Health Plan (HCHP) outcomes research, 67–68, 69; overview of outcomes research studies, 59–60, 68–69; physician involvement in TQM, 215–224, 230–260; ulcer disease, 87. See also Transurethral prostatectomy (TURP)
Centers for Disease Control and Prevention (CDC), 272
Chassin, M. R., 168
Clinical Efficacy Assessment Project, 276–277
Clinical practice: barriers to introducing TQM in, 293–301; clinical decision making versus industrial decision making, 46–48, 52–53, 296–299; total quality management (TQM)

and, 186–199; quality of care and, 83–86; randomized controlled clinical trials (RCTs) and, 182–184, 187; small area variation analysis (SAVA), 167–168, 169; sources of, 75–76, 178–182; total quality management (TQM) and, 288–289; values, preferences, and controlling variation, 94–96. *See also* Breast cancer; Coronary artery disease; Outcomes research; Transurethral prostatectomy (TURP)

W

Wadsworth, H. M., 31
Wennberg, J. E., 14, 167–168, 178, 184–185
White, W. B., 145

Z

Zimmerman, S. M., 157–158